SLIM *the* GUIDE

SLIM *the* GUIDE

For Valerie Johnson
Best wishes,
Monty Bassett

MONTY BASSETT

GREYSTONE
BOOKS
Douglas & McIntyre
Vancouver/Toronto

Copyright © 1993 by Monty Bassett
93 94 95 96 97   5 4 3 2 1

All rights reserved. No part of this book may be reproduced or transmitted in any form or by any means without permission in writing from the publisher, except by reviewers, who may quote brief passages in a review.

Greystone Books
A division of Douglas & McIntyre Ltd.
1615 Venables Street
Vancouver, British Columbia V5L 2H1

Canadian Cataloguing in Publication Data

Bassett, Monty
  Slim, the guide

  ISBN 1-55054-130-7

  I. Title.
PS8553.A77S6 1993   C813.'54   C93-091597-6
PR9199.3.B37S6 1993

Editing by Jennifer Glossop
Cover design by Jim Skipp
Cover painting of Slim Bassett by Conrad Schwiering, © the
  Estate of Mary Ethel Schwiering and Conrad Schwiering
Text design by Fiona MacGregor
Typeset by Vancouver Desktop Publishing Centre
Printed and bound in Canada by Best Gagné Book Manufacturers
Printed on acid-free paper ∞

To Agnes for her continual encouragement;
my wife, Keith Carter, for her patience and support;
Nicole, Samara and Marley for providing the reason to write,
and, most of all, to the memory of Slim, Mabel and Grover
for the stories.

CONTENTS

PREFACE ix

TRUDY'S TIME 1

SLIM, THE GUIDE 12

THE ARM 25

KATIE HAYNES 45

THE CLIMB 59

CLOUD LAKE 70

SHOEING ON THE SABBATH 86

SATURDAY NIGHT 98

CLOWNS 119

TENN 133

COLLARING ABDUL 148

WITHOUT A TRACE 157

IN SEARCH OF A SADDLE 172

PREFACE

WHEN I WAS A YOUNG MAN LIVING ON MY FOLKS' RANCH NEAR Jackson, Wyoming, storytelling was our evening entertainment. And because ours was a guest ranch, the stories we heard were about everything from million-dollar business deals made in the bloom of 1950s prosperity to trail tales told by ragged range riders on the shirt tails of a passing era.

Among the storytellers were Dr. W. H. Werkmeister, a writer and philosophy professor who came to the ranch year after year in search of the Platonic ideal of trout fishing, and John L. Lewis, the infamous United Mine Workers' boss, who—although his bodyguard actually shot the elk—gave my grandpa a "Chicago special" (a sawed-off 410 shotgun with a pistol grip) as a present. There were also people like Conrad Schwiering, the artist who painted the portrait of Grandpa on the cover of this book, and Jack Davis, a cowboy whose eyes were the bluest in the world from sitting downwind of more campfires than anyone else alive—or so he claimed. For six months of the year, Jack would guide the fat-cats and decision makers of the world (among them, Theodore Roosevelt and John D. Rockefeller) through the Teton Mountains, then in the fall he would ride all the way to southern Mexico to winter with Señora Davis and a half dozen *Davistos*. It took him six weeks each way—a forty- to fifty-day commute to work, twice a year.

Our ranch was also a way station on the tumbleweed trail for cowboys left over from the cattle-drive days. They were desperate men, looking for an audience in a world turned deaf to the men they used to be—or maybe, as Grandma said, they were just looking for a place to die.

Slim, the Guide is not their stories. Nor is it my family's history. For although my paternal grandfather was named Slim, and my father had but one arm, my family, the mountains of Wyoming and the northern Canadian wilderness are merely the seeds of fact sown on the fertile soil of imagination. What I hoped to capture in this book was the timeless wisdom of people like Slim, Ethel, Casey and Jep, for that is the one thing that remains constant in a world that has changed so drastically in the last few decades. In a single lifetime, we have altered the evolutionary course of every living organism on earth. And suddenly the slave of nature has become its master, and all that holds our power in check are our ancestors' voices of morality and self-restraint. The purpose of *Slim, the Guide* is to give volume to the insights, philosophy and humour of those voices.

TRUDY'S TIME

BUDDY LAY SPREAD-EAGLE, BAKING IN THE SPRING SUNSHINE, inhaling the smell of oven-fresh grass and yeasty sage. Resurrection Ridge, birth from death—the first place in the whole valley stretching west to the Rockies and east to the desert to spring from the snow cover. The ridge was the first tangible proof that the war with winter was over, another season of solitude survived. Resurrection of the will, Buddy hoped. He couldn't face another year like the last, what with his grandmother's death and worrying about Slim while trying to stay afloat in his first university year. But maybe that had passed with the season, and the worst was behind.

Slim, Buddy's paternal grandfather, squatted beside him on the knoll, folded up like a jackknife and balanced effortlessly on his haunches. (Buddy asked him once why he didn't sit on the ground like everyone else. "It's a habit I picked up pushing cattle in Texas," he told Buddy. "You see, in Texas, there's more cactus than chairs.") Slim noticed that the stub of the hand-rolled cigarette anchored in the side of his mouth had gone out, and he fished a wooden match from his shirt pocket. He tried to snap its head with his thumbnail, but his hands shook too much. Frustrated, he lit it on the hard heel of his boot.

The flame, sheltered in his cupped hands, exposed the recesses of deep canyons etched by years of squinting through thick trail dust and stabbing gales. His eyes grew thin, shielding out the sun reflected off the surrounding snow. Like sentries behind slits in a bunker, his eyes watched the horses on the other side of the river.

Somehow, Buddy's grandfather always knew when the

horses would make their move. The ridge was like a magnet to the herd, drawing them each year to challenge the river's high water for the first taste of green vegetation on the other side. The crossing was always dangerous, but this year an unusually heavy snowfall over the winter, plus a sudden explosion of warm weather, had swollen the river well above high-water line. Great chunks of dislodged slab ice had cascaded down the current's treacherous course, taking out the ice bridge to the horse meadow. The horses had been without hay for a week since the washout. There was still plenty of feed under the snow, but they had to paw to get it, which most of the horses did. Only the impatient ones like Slim's horse, Trudy, seriously considered Resurrection Ridge and the new green grass.

She was a tall, big-boned, chestnut-coloured thoroughbred quarter-horse cross. As far as Buddy knew, Slim was the only person ever to ride her. Slim always sat straight in the saddle, the reins in his left hand close to his chest, the mare stepping proud with her head up and an arch in her neck. Slim used to joke she had five gaits: "Start, stumble, fall, get up and go on." In truth, she could outwalk any horse on the ranch over deadfall or rockslide. "She can navigate at night down a canyon so dark you can't see your hand in front of you," Slim would say. "I do believe she smells the trail like a hunting hound!"

Slim pointed to the opposite bank, towards the procession of horses. "Trudy's bound and determined to come across," he said.

Buddy watched as the mare, in the lead, threaded her way among the willows and boulders, searching for a crossing, watching upstream for a pause in the slab ice.

"You see what's gonna happen to that damn old fool, don't you?" Slim shook his head in anticipation.

The mare had walked out on an ice ledge undercut by the river. Suddenly it collapsed with her weight, causing Trudy to scramble back to shore, spooking the other horses. Like startled kids, a few galloped wildly up the bank to the meadow, nipping and kicking at each other with fanciful fright.

"There's a lot of ice out there in the current," Slim muttered. "If a horse gets caught in it, there'll be hell to pay!"

Reaching absently into the front pocket of his wool jacket, he retrieved a pouch of Bull Durham rolling tobacco. Plunging two fingers down the throat of the sack, Slim spread the opening, then brushed off his fingers on his shirt. Holding the drawstring in his teeth, he peeled off a rolling paper and creased it into a trough. Next he shook a line of amber flakes across the paper, folded the bottom edge over the tobacco with his thumb and forefingers and began rolling from the middle towards the ends. After running his tongue along the gummed edge, he gave it a final roll.

Buddy realized the ritual hadn't changed a step over the years, only the hands that performed it. Once strong and supple, they were now lean, knobby branches covered with mottled leather. The two fingers holding the cigarette had turned a dark mahogany with years of nicotine. Once capable of making bullet-tight cigarettes on a horse in a headwind, the hands now trembled in the slightest breeze, creating loose confetti rolls that spewed a gentle shower of sparks onto Slim's wool shirt.

"Ethel used to worry we'd go broke keeping me in tobacco," the old man said, amused. It pleased Buddy to hear him talk so. It was the first time since the funeral he'd spoken of her. "Course," Slim said, smiling and studying the smoke curling from the end of the cigarette, "Ethel used to worry that even the price of pine cones would put us into Bumsville!" Again he chuckled. "Mind you, your grandmammy made a science of worrying. She'd come up with natural catastrophes even the Lord Almighty hadn't considered." He paused for a moment, reflecting. "Truth be known, we *didn't* have two coins to rub together when we first set out. Maybe that's why we got on together . . . blind necessity."

"Tell me again how you met Grandma?" Buddy pressed him, sensing the old man wanted to talk.

Slim's face winced, then rekindled with a kinder memory. "It was at a barn dance, over near Skyline. Buddy, you should've seen her! Her hair was the colour of a fawn's coat and naturally curly so it hung in ringlets around her face. And her eyes"—he pinched off a few blades of grass— "they were just this green!"

He twirled the grass with his fingers. "As soon as I seen her, I stepped right up and told her she was the prettiest woman in nineteen states and four provinces! And I weren't stretching it a bit, son! I'd been all around the country working hither 'n' yon, and I meant just what I said!"

"What did *she* say?"

"She looked me over real close." He smiled to himself, then shook his head. "And darned if she don't start laughing—not huffy like, but free like a meadowlark. I weren't sure which way to flop, whether to run or stay put, so I asked her to marry me instead!"

"Well?"

"Well! She said flat out that she wasn't going to raise a bunch of kids behind a herd of cows and a saddle tramp—thinking that'd put a stop to me.

"But I told her I had my plans. 'Sure,' I said, 'I got a saddle—but I ain't on the tramp!' She never was the best judge of character, and I had to hang around about a year or so until she seen for herself what a right fine fellow I was. Then when I asked her again, you know what she said? She says she'll do it just to stop me from pestering her!" Slim's laugh was full and open. "Can you imagine the likes? Still, I sure wasn't going to let the moment pass, so I borrowed a buckboard off the postmaster and we went over the pass to Idaho, to a cousin of Ethel's who was a prairie preacher."

"Where did you go for your honeymoon?"

"Weren't much of a honeymoon, just one day. Ethel had to get back to the hotel where she worked, and I was riding range for the Flag Ranch." Slim paused, staring at the river. "Course, some might say our whole life was our honeymoon! Son, we shared everything, decisions, hard times—everything—the marriage was a partnership.

"But we were as opposite as night and day!" Slim said. "She was a raving Republican and I'm a damn Democrat!"

Buddy suspected that since neither voted, nor cared much about politics, they were simply different sides of the same coin. Fifty-three years they pooled their energies to raise a family among the mountains of the Palmer Valley, where snow depths sometimes reached eight feet and the roads were closed more than open. Yet somehow each hardship, each crisis, just seemed to strengthen the weld between Slim and Ethel.

Sandwiched between two large boulders, Trudy and a big

buckskin gelding were shouldering each other for the lead like two polo ponies in a ride off.

"Did I ever tell you how I come by Trudy?" Slim asked.

At least a dozen times, thought Buddy, but the story was one of his favourites; besides, as Slim claimed, he could tell a story ten times and never rewalk the same path.

"I got her as a foal," Slim said, nodding towards Trudy, who'd taken the lead from the buckskin. "I could tell right off that she had a good measure of character by the way she pranced around her mammy." He shook his head. "But, boy-howdy! I didn't figure on quite so much!

"Started handling her as a yearling, saddling her, picking up her feet and all. But it weren't till she was a four-year-old that I finally got around to giving her a try with a saddle. I figured she'd throw a tizzy fit, so I snubbed her up with a short rein till I had a deep seat. And, sure enough, the second I slacked off, it was Katie bar the door!"

He stopped to strike a match on his zipper. Taking a long puff that produced a fresh lava stream of sparks, he blew out the match, rolled the head between his thumb and index finger, then flipped it towards the embankment.

"When she cut loose, she fired straight up! Just like one of them Roman candles. In fact, I figured she was gonna rear over backwards, so I kicked loose a stirrup, fixing to step clear, but, don't you know, she ups and pitches forward instead! Sent me rolling across the corral like a billiard ball.

"In those days I fancied myself a pretty fair rider so I got back on her right away, thinking she'd just got in a lucky shot. And the next time when she comes up high like she'd done before, I stayed put and we hit the ground hard enough to near punch my feet through my boots. But she don't waste no slack mourning my hurt before she takes off for the sky again, and this time she throws a twist in her tail and does a sunfish fandango that sets me to going one way while she's cutting the other." Slim clapped his hands, laughing. "I plowed more dust that afternoon than most prairie farmers do in a year."

To Buddy's thinking, Trudy never was completely broken. Certainly not her spirit. Predictably, each spring she'd test Slim. Once, Buddy crept down to the corral early in the morning to watch them. Slim swung into the saddle and immediately the horse humped up. "What ails you, you ol' fool?" he barked. "Now step out smartly!" He brought his heels against her ribs, not hard, but it was enough to provoke Trudy. Buddy had never seen a horse buck so high or hard. His grandpa stayed with her, but, oh, what a beating he took to do it. Still, when the annual event was over, Trudy didn't buck again—until the next spring.

"I never understood why you put up with the punishment. I would have sold that horse long ago," Buddy said.

Slim looked at him, astonished. "Buddy, you can't go along in life just taking the mounts that suit you. Pretty soon you'd be walking more than you're riding. 'Sides, a horse with any gumption is going to stand up to you, right?" Slim paused for a moment. "I guess it depends on how you want to go. You want to ride in style, you gotta pay the price!"

"I guess I'm just a De Soto car man." Buddy sighed and laid back on the grass. The sun was directly overhead, much too full for philosophy. "Wake me if there's an Indian attack." He closed his eyes.

"Or stampling horses?"

"You still think they'll try crossing today?"

"Bet your bottom dollar on it!"

Stampling horses! Buddy was shocked when he went away to school to discover he knew more words than Webster's dictionary. *Stample*, a merger of *stampede* and *trample*; usage: "Poor thing was stampled!" Or *yon*—most people thought it was something you did when you were tired. They didn't know it was the place just behind hither. Buddy also discovered, that first year of school, that beyond encyclopedia facts and figures, everything he knew of fundamental importance he'd learned from Slim.

Lessons were catch as catch can: studying tracks in the soft mud around a mineral lick or firewood philosophizing while splitting pine on a chopping block. The classes Buddy remembered best were the evenings on the back porch off the kitchen. Twilight, after supper and chores, he and Slim would sit there watching Palmer Peak turn lavender with the sunset. Sometimes, while his grandpa studied the peak for mountain sheep, he'd let Buddy try rolling from the Bull Durham pouch. Usually the boy produced blimps, swollen with tobacco in the middle and the ends twisted too tight for the smoke to pass. "You sure we're related?" Slim would tease him. People didn't come more related. Even Buddy's name mirrored that. His parents christened him Alexander, but Slim judged it too highfalutin for such a little tadpole, so he evolved through a lineage of nicknames. Following Tadpole came Skeezix, after a newspaper comic character. Then there was Gizzy-wibet, a word of Slim's invention for that age when kids love to be kidded, and reason and the ridiculous hold no difference. Finally, about the time the boy could sit a horse well enough to keep up with him, Slim settled upon Buddy. Reasoning it was the best one yet, even his parents accepted the title.

The back-porch lessons came in many ways: hooting for an owl until it landed on the gable above them or side-aching laughter at calamities that only hours before had scared the hell out of them. Like the time they got ledged up on Palmer Peak with a sheep hunter, a business executive from Albany, New York. "I learned something today," Buddy's grandfather said to the hunter that evening as they sat on the back porch looking at the ledge through binoculars. "Makes no never mind if a person's a millionaire or a hillbilly. In the mountains we's all on equal footing"—then he grinned a big barrel-slat grin—"which generally ain't that solid!"

Sometimes the lessons were subtle, their significance not surfacing for years, seeds sown for a future harvest. And sometimes they were stark and immediate, like the elk over on Boulder Creek.

Buddy and Slim had come upon this crippled bull elk near the Boulder Creek trail. Actually, they heard it first, a horrible sucking and gurgling sound. Somebody had gutshot it through the rib cage. Its lungs were full of blood, and a crimson froth bubbled around the puncture like soapsuds. Judging by the blood matted across the ground, the elk had been thrashing around for some time before finally falling downhill and wedging itself helplessly against a small spruce. Slim was off Trudy with his .348 rifle before Buddy even knew what was happening.

It was probably the rifle report that alerted Chauncey Fenton and his two boys. Before Slim and Buddy had finished dressing out the animal, they rode up.

"Slim!" Fenton yelled. "That's my elk."

Buddy's grandfather didn't say a word, just stood there staring at Fenton. "If you reckon," he finally said, quietly, "come take him."

Buddy was scared. He could feel his grandpa's rage. But Fenton, not given to perception of subtleties, rode closer with a cock-of-the-walk grin. Slim was on Fenton like a cougar, seizing him by the coat and jerking him from his horse. He gave Fenton a shove with his boot, driving the guy headlong. Fenton hit the dead elk running and fell forward onto the bloody carcass. Buddy's eyes darted to the Fenton boys. Neither moved. Immediately Fenton was on his feet. There was elk blood smeared across his face and the front of his down jacket. He clenched his fists and started for Slim.

"Mister"—Slim's tone was measured and level—"I'd think twice about that." Buddy knew if Fenton pressed him further, Slim wouldn't stop with just a beating. Fenton must have felt it, too.

"I shamed myself today," Slim said that evening as they hung the last quarter of elk in the cooler. "I shouldn't have given a no count like of Fenton the benefit of my anger. But, son, there's no greater evil on earth than causing suffering unnecessarily. Everything has a right to a quick death!"

Few things angered Slim, but he had no patience for anyone who didn't respect *Her*. If he had a religion at all, it was a simple faith in Mother Nature. It was a faith fuelled by the mountains, but instead of prayer and penance, Slim practised his faith with admiration and amazement. Even dressing out game was a mixture of science and sacrament for Slim. "Look here, Buddy," he'd say to the boy, pointing out the individual chambers of a heart. "Ain't that something how all them muscles can work just fine together! And do it time and again without missing a beat! Even our De Soto can't match that!"

Respect. Buddy guessed that was why Slim and Ethel lived in peace with the land and themselves. But the land changed without their realizing it. And while they sat unaware on the porch watching a much slower clock, a cycle measured by generations of elk and mountain sheep feeding across the slopes of Palmer Peak, roads like weed roots began creeping into the valley from the sides. Gradually more and more of the once self-sustaining wilderness fell under the control of managers—wildlife managers, forest managers. "Manure managers." His grandpa lumped them together and gave them little attention, maybe hoping natural predation would eventually eliminate the nuisance. Unfortunately, Slim had underestimated the army of bureaucrats and failed to see that soon there would be more managers than the animals they managed.

Time was no more kind to Buddy's grandparents. Slim's years in the saddle began taking their toll, his legs becoming crippled and withered from poor circulation. Then the retina in one eye was partially torn when a young colt Buddy should have been riding (Slim was sixty and Buddy was sixteen at the time) bucked down a rockslide. His grandmother's health never was good: diabetes, high blood pressure and a beaver's addiction to work. Then, just when Slim and Ethel were ready to retire and turn the ranch over to Buddy's parents, Ethel died of a heart attack.

Slim was lost. In the middle of the night Buddy would hear him moving around the ranch house. From his bedroom window Buddy saw the old man's dark form limping awkwardly down the hill to the corral. Faintly there'd come a whistle. "Step out smartly, mare," Buddy imagined Slim saying as he reined Trudy away from the saddle shed. Then, like fleeting phantoms, they'd disappear into the night. Dread consumed the boy in those vacant hours. He felt helpless, groundless. He'd never suspected there could be a limit to Slim's courage.

Through those eternal nights Buddy lay awake, imagining what he'd say to his grandfather when he returned . . . *if* he returned. "You've no right," was Buddy's first thought. But why not? Wasn't it Slim's right to choose his death? In fact, Slim made a joke, which Buddy had always sensed was more than a joke. "If I ever get so gimped I can't fend on my own, just soak me in honey and tether me somewhere for bear bait— might as well get some use out of my miserable remains!"

Buddy's grandfather had had a life envied by many men though lived by very few people. Bedridden, senile—for a man like Slim, that would be worse than death itself. Eventually Buddy's thoughts always came back to the crippled elk on Boulder Creek.

The worst of it was, Buddy realized, even if he could find the words, he was afraid to confront Slim. His grandpa, for all his qualities, was an insular man. And for all they shared, Buddy suddenly saw that there was still a great distance separating them. Fortunately, Trudy always found her way home, and at dawn she'd faithfully return with her rider.

"*Now* what ails you, you ol' fool?" The alarm in Slim's voice snapped Buddy from his reverie. His grandfather was on his feet, shielding his eyes with his hands and looking intently at the river. Immediately Buddy saw what was happening. Trudy had waded too far into the water, and its force swept her off her feet. Desperately, the mare tried to swim upstream, but the current swung her around. She held her head high, her nostrils flared, as she fought the river. Her eyes were wild. A sandbar jutted out on their side of the river. Trudy tried to reach it, but a thick slab of floating ice slammed against her, turning her downstream. She lunged, and the block of ice rolled across her back, momentarily pinning her beneath the surface. When she came up again, she'd been swept far beyond the sandbar, and the shoreline was steep and lined with large boulders. Still determined, Trudy swam until she'd breached the mainstream. Finally, caught in a back eddy, she pulled towards the rocky bank. Scrambling, she pulled herself out of the water.

"She did it!" Buddy yelled. "She damn well did it!"

His grandfather was silent for some time, watching the horse. "She ain't home yet," he said. "Look there, at her hindquarters. Something ain't right."

At first Buddy didn't see it, then he realized her back end was slowly sagging. She collapsed onto her haunches, balancing for a moment, before going completely limp and falling into the river. There was no fight left, and her head went under.

Both men stood motionless. Buddy knew the horse was dead before her head hit the water, a heart attack, he guessed. Yet desperately he hoped for some sign of life. The moments stretched, but the animal didn't move. Then Buddy went cold. Slim was no longer beside him!

Slowly, deliberately, the old man walked towards the cliff.

Buddy ran for his grandfather, catching him just before the hard edge gave way to loose shale. His frame felt frail in Buddy's grip, bones and leather. Buddy was ashamed: he'd never challenged his grandfather before. Gently he turned Slim, afraid of the reproach he'd find in the old man's eyes. Instead they were hollow like empty wells reaching far into the earth. The strength and passion were gone, and Buddy saw just how deeply grief had ravaged Slim.

"Oh, Christ!" Buddy blurted. His voice cracked. He closed his eyes to fight the tears. The arguments weighed on those eternal nights came rushing back, but again they seemed weak, unconvincing. "Maybe it is Trudy's time, but she fought it right to the end," Buddy wanted to say, but the words wouldn't come.

Then suddenly anger gripped him. "Damn you!" He shook Slim hard. "You can't do this to me! I still need you!" He searched Slim's face. "Look at me!" Buddy cried.

The chiselled features, a mask cut in stone, betrayed no response. It was over; Buddy released his grip. He could do no more. He felt humiliated for his weakness, for his anger and disrespect. Again he closed his eyes, his mind. He wanted no memories of that moment.

But then he sensed something in Slim, a slight seismic shift far down in the core of the old man. Very slowly, the grey granite mask became flush again with blood, and Slim drew himself erect. He stared at Buddy with a soft and liquid look that Buddy had never seen. Then his eyes reached beyond Buddy, to the river downstream. Already the current had moved the horse's body, forcing it into a logjam.

"Damn ol' fool." Although Slim's voice came from a great distance, it once again had body. "She never did have a lick of patience." His mottled hand reached out to Buddy for balance. Together they moved back from the cliff.

SLIM, THE GUIDE

"THE MOTHER'S FULL WITH CHILD," THE YOUNG MAN MUSED AS he studied the peaks lining the divide. Their cornices sagged heavy with the spring snow, like milk-swollen breasts over a pregnant belly. It was going to be a hot day; the breast could only get heavier. Soon the avalanches would break off, closing the mountain pass until June. Slim was counting on that. He turned his binoculars down the valley, to the dark, featureless figure moving steadily across the white blanket. For two days Slim had been waiting, but now it was over.

He returned the binoculars to their case and began packing his Spartan camp onto the bent-poplar pack frame. Taking some snow on the end of his mitt, he rubbed clean his single cook pot and stuffed it with small leather bags of salt, coffee and jerky. Setting aside his pistol, he crushed his bedroll against his chest and rolled it around a thin willow branch, like a tight scroll. Then, pulling out the branch, he lashed the bedroll to his pack frame. Finally, he folded up the tarp he'd used for a windbreak over his snow-pit shelter and covered the load with it.

For some time, Slim knelt against his pack looking at the pistol. It was a big, heavy Colt revolver, .45 caliber with enough wallop to stop an angry sow bear. But the recoil caused the barrel to lift, making it hard to shoot accurately— he'd have to use both hands. It was obvious the gun was government issue; the bluing was flawless like polished plate. A cowboy's Colt would be scratched and freckled with beads of rust and trail dust. Slim imagined a clerk in the fish and game office, desk-bound by job and choice, tending to the pistol with loving care and dreams of shooting poachers between their thieving eyes. Slim wondered how much he would have to use the pistol. A few pelts weren't worth killing a man over, that was for sure—probably not even worth crippling him. Besides, if Slim wounded the guy, what would he do then, drag the poacher all the way to Skyline through the belly-deep snow? No, Slim decided, the pistol should be the last resort.

Of course, Moose Tooth didn't have to know this. As long as he *thought* Slim would use the Colt, Slim might never have to use it. On the other hand, it was likely the poacher had a rifle, and Slim wasn't anxious to get shot just because he was afraid to use his gun. He had to get the upper hand on the trapper and hold it through to the end. Picking up the pistol, he checked the cylinder, assuring himself it was loaded, then he dropped it in the pocket of his Mackinaw.

Slim stood up with his pack on. He was a tall, gangly young man with large, knobby features on an ascetic frame. "Knots along a length of rope," his mother used to tell him. His face was linear, with a high forehead and a forged chin set on a sharp, dog-leg jaw line. His nose, once thin and fine, had been broken and spread wide at the bridge, crowding his sage-grey eyes, adding to their inscrutability. It was Slim's mouth that betrayed his character. It was wide and expressive, and even when it turned down, it turned up.

Hunched over and kicking the tips of his snowshoes forward, he moved along the long shadows of tall spruce towards the edge of the clearing and the dwarfed fir skirting the sides of the narrow valley. In the shadows his tracks wouldn't show, but in the open sun they'd stand out like flags. Finally he reached the snow crater under the last clump of fir before the open meadow. Keeping his webs on, he rolled under the trees and into the snow pit, flopping against the wall facing the clearing. There he waited, breathing into his mitt so the vapour of his breath wouldn't betray his hiding place.

"Moose Tooth!" Slim sang out when the black dot grew into a man bent beneath the weight of a great pack, which, Slim suspected, was mainly furs.

"You got company!" Slim yelled, pleased with the way the surrounding rock cliffs added tenor and authority to his voice.

Mr. Tooth probably thinks the Lord Almighty has come to collect. Slim laughed to himself.

Recovering from his shock, the trapper dropped his pack in the snow and, with one swift movement, swung his rifle to his shoulder. But he couldn't locate the source of the call.

"Mister, don't mistake me. I'll kill you if I have to," Slim warned, wrapping his fingers around the Colt in his pocket. His chest felt tight; his heart began to race. If he was going to have to use the gun, now would be the time. "Put your rifle down on the pelts!" he commanded, trying to hold the fear from his voice.

Moose Tooth stood motionless. He looked in Slim's direction but, caught by the blinding sun, didn't seem to have a fix on Slim. Slim guessed the trapper was weighing his alternatives. Out in the open, he couldn't make a run for it, not on webs. Besides, the poacher wouldn't know how many of them there were. Reluctantly, Moose finally laid down the carbine.

Slim climbed out of the snow well and walked cautiously towards the trapper, stopping just a few yards from the man. His hand still gripped the Colt in his pocket. "That looks plumb silly!" Slim smiled, pointing to the snowshoes Moose Tooth wore backwards and to the poles the trapper had used for lifting their tails as he walked forward on them. "But it sure is smart!" Slim laughed so easily that even the trapper momentarily smiled. "However, I bet you'll find the walk to Skyline a lot easier if you turned them around."

The poacher was obviously surprised that Slim was alone. He eyed him closely, as though assessing his chances to grab his rifle or maybe jump Slim and try to overpower him.

Slim just grinned. It kept his teeth from chattering. And he waited. It was like waiting to see which way a startled grizzly would go, whether he'd run from you—or at you. With his hand still in his pocket, he pointed the Colt's barrel at the trapper's stomach. Then he saw it—the resignation in the trapper's eyes. Slim would have no more trouble with him.

The trapper grunted as he knelt and reversed his snowshoes so they faced forward.

Slim had seen the trapper before. His features were unforgettable: his hatchet nose, the ladle-round cheekbones, his illusive, anthracite eyes that seemed to see everything but projected little back. The Indian reminded Slim of a granite ledge—solid and impassive, smooth and polished by time and the elements. But judging by the tracks of errant tobacco encrusted in the corners of his mouth and the yellowing on his teeth, the Indian was not alien to the white man's habits. Then Slim noticed it. The trapper's incisors were quite ordinary! From his nickname, Slim had always figured Moose Tooth would have a set of teeth that could strip a poplar without touching the bark with his lips.

Moose Tooth stood and started to sling his pack onto his back, but Slim stopped him.

"Here," Slim said, "I'll take the pelts. I ain't carrying an owl's hoot, and you seem to have a load. Besides, I guess now they're my responsibility, ain't they?" He took the skins and tied them to his own pack frame.

Then he picked the carbine off the snow. And, working the lever action, he chambered a live cartridge into the barrel. "A loaded rifle ain't safe, you know." He grinned, locking his eyes onto the trapper's. "Ready?"

Moose Tooth looked puzzled.

Blam! Blam! Blam! He fired the rifle into the air three times in rapid succession.

Nothing! Nothing, except echo upon echo of the rifle reports ascending through the pass.

Blam! He shot again into the air and waited. Then, just as he prepared to fire the last round, he felt the earth give a slight, almost imperceptible sigh.

Whumph! It was a dull sound, like someone punching a pillow, and for that brief second, the entire valley seemed to exhale, then hold its breath in silence. Suddenly, the monster that had been growing through the winter, harbouring the fury of countless blizzards and savage winds, sprang free. Roaring, bellowing, snapping off trees and grinding them to spears and splinters, the jaws of the avalanche crushed and chewed everything in its reach. Voracious winds, full of thick, suffocating snow, raced over the slope ahead of the slide. Boiling across the valley bottom, the violent winds slammed into the opposite wall of the divide. Again the tenuous balance of snow and rock snapped, and again cornices collapsed, triggering more avalanches. And soon a chain reaction started across the pass, as slides provoked slides, until the entire mountain valley shook with their thunder. The sun turned dark and evil behind the great cloud of snow. Both men stood transfixed, mesmerized—terrified.

Then it happened. Over the mammoth roar, they heard the burden on the peak above them break loose.

"Run!" yelled the trapper, though not moving himself.

Slim lunged forward to escape, but his feet held fast. The snow had compacted like concrete around his snowshoes. Suddenly the wind slammed him face first onto the hard crust, knocking the breath out of him. He gasped, but the air had substance. He gagged, desperately pulling his hands to his face and pushing open a pocket in front of his mouth.

Then there was silence. Slim didn't know how long he'd lain there—maybe only a moment, though a moment he thought would never end. Maybe it didn't; maybe he was dead. No, he decided, he could hear his breathing and feel his heart throbbing. Maybe the slide hadn't hit him after all. Cautiously, he moved an arm, discovering little resistance. Slowly, he arched back, finding only a few inches of wind-drifted powder snow covering him. His feet were still buckled to the webs, which were still anchored to the crust. His right knee burned from the fall forward, but as he cautiously moved it, it didn't seem broken. It could have been worse, he decided, much worse.

Slim looked around for the trapper. With his mitt, he pushed an adjacent hummock of snow. It pushed back. Gingerly the trapper lifted himself away from the snow and looked around with wide, unbelieving eyes.

Where only moments before the pass had bellowed with unholy apocalypse, a monastic peace held the land. A thin cloud of snow dust hung lightly above the valley, settling like fine-sifted flour. Except for the occasional slab of perimeter snow breaking loose and slipping down the gouged-out chutes, nothing moved. But the scar ran from rim rock to rim rock. Nothing was left untouched. Even on the steep pine ridges, like the one above them, which had deflected the avalanche away from the men, the trees were snapped off thirty to forty feet above the ground by the ferocious winds as though sliced down by a great sickle.

Suddenly, to Slim's astonishment, Moose let out a loud, joyous yell. Raising his arms skyward, he started to dance, jigging up and down on one leg then the other, though his feet were still strapped to his inert webs. Slim understood. Everywhere around them had been hit. Had he intercepted Moose Tooth just a few minutes earlier, or even fifty yards farther up the trail, they would have been crushed beneath tons of snow boulders.

Then, just as abruptly as Moose had begun dancing, he stopped. His dark eyes narrowed as he looked straight at Slim. There was no mistaking their question.

Slim shrugged. "Well, my plan was just to close your escape route over into Idaho," he said. Then, looking at the snow barricading the valley around them, he added sheepishly, "I guess I got a little ambitious, huh?"

The trapper studied Slim. Finally, he shook his head with disbelief. "You ain't so smart as I tho't." He gave a heavy sigh, then bending over and still shaking his head, he began digging his snowshoes from the hard-packed snow.

It took the rest of the morning and most of the afternoon to cross the avalanche field separating them from Skyline. Their webs were useless on the vaulted boulders of snow. The spikes of splintered trees, sticking out like quills on a porcupine, threatened to shred their snowshoes' leather lacing. Slim had never seen anything like it. It seemed as though a great egg-beater had scrambled rock, sod and vegetation into an icing mix, then spread it helter-skelter across the valley. When the slides melted, pockets of rich, black topsoil would form from the rotting mass, and new forests would grow from the scarified cones. Nature tilling the soil, Slim thought, then laughed, remembering that he had had a role in the event.

It became obvious, when they finally reached the other side of the avalanche sweep, that they wouldn't make it to Skyline that night. Also, Slim's leg was starting to go numb from the searing fire of the torn tendons. They'd have to lay over at the Wilson cabin and go on the next day.

The cabin wasn't much, a pole-and-sod shack all but buried beneath twelve-foot snowdrifts. They had to dig down to reach the door, which fortunately opened inward. Inside there was a barrel stove, a plank table impregnated with moss and lichen, and two cots against the north wall. The cross rafters sagged so low that the men had to hunch over to keep from striking their heads. The trapper scrounged some dry limbs off the pine trees outside, and soon Slim had a pot of water boiling. He added some of his jerky and the rice that Moose Tooth was carrying. On a ledge above the door, Slim found two stubby tallow candles.

"How'd you'd come by the name Moose Tooth?" Slim asked, standing over the pot on the stove.

The Indian reached inside his deerskin shirt and drew out a necklace made of teeth, dozens of moose teeth strung together on a leather thong.

"My name's Jep . . . Jep Cashaw, t'at's my name." Then he looked at Slim. "You's ta saddle tramp from Flag Ranch, ain't you? I seen you last summer when I packs t'em government men up ta Buffalo River."

"They call me Slim." He extended his hand to the Indian. "And you're part right, the Buffalo's where I seen you, too. But you're dead wrong about the saddle tramp. I'm a man with a future. And, don't forget, Jep Cashaw"—Slim's eyes twinkled in the candlelight—"I'm also the man that caught you."

"Takes you long enough," Jep growled. "Four winters."

"No, it didn't! That was the other fellers. It took *me* only three days. One to figure out what you were up to and two more to get to where you were going."

"How you knows?" Jep asked.

"Your tracks. See, normally the heel of a snowshoe digs in first, then it drags out a little tail when it moves forwards. But yours didn't. Instead, the *front* of your shoe pulled across the track." Slim pushed the palm of his hand down and pulled it forward. "Them other fellers figured you'd left the valley, when all along you were right under their noses. And when they thought they was following you, they was really getting farther away!

"I found your tracks along the river, and when I seen what you was up to, I just followed them backwards till I was sure of where you were going." Slim grinned.

"But 'ow you knows t'at?" Jep stared at Slim, still puzzled.

"Like hunting elk. If you go to where they are, they'll already be gone by the time you get there. But if you go where they's *going*, they'll come to you— just like you come to me." Again Slim smiled. "Besides, it weren't no mystery that you'd be going over to Idaho to sell your furs. That's where the price is best—and there ain't but one pass open in the winter. I figured by the time you'd checked your last trap set, I'd be there waiting."

Jep sat for a long time brooding. "Slim, t'ey's gone too far," he said finally. "Ain't ta land of ta free." He spat tobacco juice towards the far corner of the cabin, away from the bunks. "Not no more. You t'ink back-time trappers like Colter needed permits to catch fur? You t'ink t'ey begs for permission?"

Slim considered his point. "In fact, they did," he argued. "They paid up just like everyone else."

Jep looked suspiciously at him, not understanding.

"Sure, if they wanted to do business in a territory for more than one season, they got permission from the local chief. Your problem is you didn't go to the chief—the government."

Jep grunted at the word *government*. "Why t'ey cares? A man works 'ard trapping. Off alone from 'is people. Easy to dies and nobody even knows—maybe an avalanche gets 'im. I say t'at man earn every skin."

"Laws and taxes, Jep, they're just some of the curses the white man's got up his sleeve." Slim stirred the soup, prodding the jerky with his knife to break it apart against the side of the pot. "The land's changing, Jep. Maybe you don't see it so much here holed up in the valley, but outside, it's all different." He looked at the trapper. "For one thing, there's a flood of folks coming west. The railroad's taking the beef out but bringing back people from the east. And I'll tell you straight, every dern one of them's got some notion of getting something free from the land. Timber, skins, crops, don't matter. And I know this for a fact, cuz I seen it myself. They've damn near trapped the Rockies down to the last tree squirrel. Fact, that's why they's paying premium for pelts nowadays. They's getting damn scarce."

"A dozen pelts ain't gonna make no difference ta no government." Jep's voice was full of anger.

"Maybe not, but a hundred fellers each thinking the same way *is* going to make a difference." Slim poked the jerky. "It ain't the change so much. It's how fast it's coming. Remember it weren't so long ago the buffalo outnumbered the prairie chickens, and now they's almost gone. Jep, there's got to be some control." Slim gave the pot a final stir and wiped his hunting knife on the rim. "Dinner is served," he announced.

Slim lay awake on his bunk, thinking about Jep. He smiled, remembering the happy dance the Indian did when he realized how close they'd come to being crushed to death. He liked Jep, and he was sorry he had to take him in. Besides, what *was* Jep's crime? Being born a hundred years too late? Hell, Slim thought, he wished *he'd* been born a century earlier. Back around the turn of the 1800s, that would be about right. Sixty years before the Yankee army "tamed" the frontier. Being a southerner, Slim never understood how the Yankees could free the slaves and then stick the Indians on reservations. Maybe the settlers should have been confined to reservations and the Indians and trappers allowed to run the land. Maybe he should just let Jep go.

Slim saw something else he shared with Jep: they were both being chased by the same avalanche. Slim knew when the trail drive broke up in Cheyenne that it was the last one for most of the riders. Maybe even the last trail drive ever. Two men had been killed on the drive, one rancher and one trail hand, in different fracases, but both over cross-fencing. Wire had drawn and quartered the open range, he realized. The West had been butchered by ownership.

Some riders had talked about quitting the saddle, going off to a sister's farm near Des Moines or Lethbridge. Sitting down under a shady tree with the nieces and nephews, telling them what great men they used to be. Others confided to Slim about a long-pampered dream, a memory of a lonely woman, maybe a teacher or a widow who'd passed through their lives when times weren't so desperate.

But Slim knew that the hard-core saddle tramps would just drift like tumbleweeds from fence line to fence line. Age and wear would eventually catch them in a slat-board shack wedged between the edge of town and the prairie. Then one day they'd simply wander out into the desert at forty below to take a pee, and never come back.

As Slim lay there looking into the dark, he thought about the desert. First it was buffalo skulls, the wind threading through their vacant sockets. Then came the skeletons of Indians, then settlers and soldiers. Next there were cattle carcasses, strays and cripples from the trail drives. Now, Slim thought, it was cowboys. Cowboys and Indians gone out to pee in minus forty degrees.

Well, Slim thought, sighing, he wasn't going to be one of them. He rolled over onto his side. He was young, he had choices and ambition and, most of all, he had Ethel.

Slim thought about Ethel. He smiled as he considered how, in a way, he was like the debris deposited by the avalanche. Fate had uprooted him from Mississippi, carried him through Mexico, Texas, Cheyenne and finally dumped him in Skyline, either to take root or to rot on the spot. Slim took root. He and Ethel had been married a year and two months. Their first child was just a few months away. They'd taken up a homestead in the Palmer Valley, and they shared a dream. Slim was still afraid it was a risky venture, but they'd decided to start a ranch for dudes. They'd guide folks from back east around the mountains; take them fishing, hunting, sightseeing. "Slim, the guide," Ethel used to tease him, but the title sat well with Slim.

Still, maybe it wasn't so risky. Slim and Ethel had learned that the men Jep had packed down the Buffalo and Yellowstone rivers were surveyors contracted by the government to lay the boundaries for a new national park. In fact, he and Ethel already had an advanced booking to take a family on a pack trip into the proposed park, three weeks in July.

Slim awoke before dawn. The pain in his leg had made his sleep fitful. He would have to leave the furs at the cabin. He couldn't ask Jep to carry them. He'd have to tie them up out of reach of the porcupines and get them when his leg was better.

"Maybe I gives you ta pelts?" Jep said in the dark cabin.

"You can't, I already got 'em."

"T'ey paying yous t' brings me in?"

"Ten dollars a day if I caught you, plus food and use of their hand-polished Colt."

"T'ose furs bring twice t'at in Idaho." Jep pressed his point.

There was a long silence as Slim considered Jep's offer. "Couldn't live with myself, now, could I?" A grin swept across Slim's face. "You being out here free as the breeze, taking the public's furs without so much as a handshake." He fell silent again. "Do you know how to pack horses?" Slim finally asked.

Jep was puzzled. "T'at's what I does comes summer."

"Well, maybe I could use a good packer this summer," Slim offered, as he rose and began building the breakfast fire. "How come you never got a permit?" he asked Jep. "They don't cost a mound of moose turds."

Jep studied the rafters, faintly lit by the small fire. "Can't read or write," he said at last.

Slim stared at Jep for some time. "Me neither," he admitted. "But maybe Ethel could teach us. She does fine with words and numbers."

As they stood in front of the new log government building, neither Slim nor Jep looked like the two men who'd straggled into Skyline the day before. Jep had had a bath, then Ethel took her scissors to his long black hair, and Slim had lent him a change of clothes. It was Ethel's idea that they should look good for the judge. Slim even put on new wool trousers, their factory crease still fresh. On a shelf he found the game warden badge that Benson, the chief warden, had given him, and pinned it on the pocket flap of his Mackinaw. "Ready?" Slim asked.

A clerk went to Benson's door to announce Slim and Jep. Probably the same clerk, Slim speculated, who'd polished the Colt in the safety of his office.

"There's someone to see you, sir."

As Slim and Jep stepped into the warden's office, the heat from the wood stove rushed past them to escape the confined room.

"I'd like you to meet Jep Cashaw," Slim said, stepping up to the polished desk.

Unsure of whom he was meeting, Benson rose and extended his hand enthusiastically to Slim's friend. Then he looked at Slim quizzically.

"And I'll take my reward money now," Slim said with a full grin.

"This is the poacher?" the fish and game officer exclaimed, astonished. "You Moose Tooth?"

"His name is Jep Cashaw."

Benson stared at him disbelievingly. The man looked like a Jep Cashaw, the warden thought—not Moose Tooth, a poacher who'd confounded some of his best wardens for four seasons. It didn't make sense. Then there was the cowboy. Showed up with no experience, and in less than a week he accomplished what Benson's trained staff couldn't do.

"Where's the evidence?" Benson asked finally, trying to regain his command of the situation. "You catch him with any evidence?"

"Half-dozen marten, about the same number of beaver and a couple mink," Slim replied.

"Well, where are they?"

"They didn't make it to town," Slim said apologetically. "My leg got bummed up in an avalanche and I just couldn't carry them any farther."

Jep just shrugged. "And *I* ain't about t'carry my own gallows, is I?"

Benson nodded for Slim to follow him down the hall to the judge's chambers. "Better watch him closely," Slim said to the clerk, pointing at Jep. "He's plum bush crazy, might try most anything. You got a gun?" The clerk's eyes darted to the prisoner, then to Slim's solemn face.

In the judge's chambers Slim explained about the capture, the avalanche, his leg injury and why the evidence was cached on the trail. The judge asked if Jep had put up any resistance.

"None at all," Slim replied.

"Well, the evidence doesn't make much difference, he's still guilty," the judge said. "But usually the fine is based on the amount of contraband they got in their possession. You say six beaver, six marten and two mink?"

"That's about right," Slim nodded.

"And how much do you owe this man?" the judge asked Benson, pointing to Slim.

"What did we agree to? Ten dollars a day? For four days," Benson calculated. "That would be forty dollars."

"Well, that isn't too out of line with the fine. I'll make the fine equal to the reward. That way the government isn't losing money," the judge decided.

When they got back to his office, Benson took four ten-dollar gold pieces from a locked cash box in his desk and handed them to Slim. Slim unpinned the badge and laid it on the table. Remembering the pistol, he retrieved it from his pocket, opened the cylinder and emptied the shells into his hand. He handed the pistol to the clerk and laid the bullets by the badge.

"Six rounds issued, six rounds returned," Slim said proudly.

Jep rose to go with Benson to the judge's chambers. Then, turning to Slim, he suddenly stuck out his hand. "I comes see you in spring 'bout t'at packing job."

"You do that," Slim said. "And it could be a spell before I get back to the Wilson cabin." He tapped his leg. "Be too bad to just let the squirrels have those furs." He smiled. "So, good luck, Jep Cashaw." Slim shook the Indian's hand. "I hope the judge ain't in a hanging mood."

The transfer of the four coins passed smoothly and unnoticed by either Benson or his clerk.

THE ARM

ETHEL STOOD IN THE DOORWAY TO THE DOCTOR'S OFFICE, holding tightly to her leather purse with one red, chapped hand while the other absently patted at the swan-wing wave of white hair framing her face. In spite of the floral-print blue dress and the practical wool Pendleton jacket she wore over it, she had a strong, stately bearing, tall and ruler straight. Not that she was proud. She stood with command because it hurt her back to do otherwise.

Resolutely, she drew a deep breath and entered the psychiatrist's office. The soft carpet that cushioned her step was a welcome relief after the hard wooden floors that thumped and groaned and made her legs tired by the end of the day. The light fragrance of lemon furniture wax was also comforting, for it meant that the doctor took care of things. On the walls there were diplomas and mountain pictures, not the specimen shelves she had feared. Ethel really didn't know what psychiatrists did, but as she looked around, she saw the office was quite ordinary: no bars on the windows, no fences or guards. Most of all, Ethel was pleased that the doctor was a woman. Ethel had so many questions about why her son had been committed, questions that she could never ask a man.

"I'm sorry to take you from the ranch with winter so close," said the doctor, coming from behind her desk to greet Ethel. "But I think it's important that we talk." She was a slender woman with her hair drawn back in a bun. Her features were delicate, yet her eyes were large and pleasant.

The doctor offered Ethel a seat on the couch and sat down beside her. "Tea?" she asked, reaching for a porcelain Chinese teapot that sat on a polished coffee table. The cup felt thin and elegant in Ethel's hands, fragile and refined in comparison to the thick, heavy, indestructible coffee mugs she was used to.

"Your son is quite a remarkable young man. I guess you know that I've taken a special interest in his case," the doctor began, "but there is still much I don't understand, and I was hoping you could tell me more about him. Particularly his childhood, and about how he lost his arm."

"I'll do what I can," Ethel said. "Lord knows I've been over it enough times myself these last four months." She studied her hands. "But the truth is, I don't have any answers."

The doctor reached over and touched Ethel's arm gently. "Don't concern yourself with answers. Why not start with your earliest memories? Often that's the easiest way to begin."

Ethel collected her thoughts. She smiled. "Casey was born to the Lord's own perfection. Two arms, two legs and a smile that could melt a glacier. He was a winter child, you know, born in February. Slim, that's my husband, always said a winter litter is the toughest, and I guess in some ways Casey is proof of the pudding. And once, all the seasons lived in that boy. He had so much fire and energy—he was going to set the world on its ear. Now,"—she sighed—"there's only winter. He's like a winter landscape, all frozen beneath a blanket of snow so that you don't see much of what's underneath. But"—she caught herself—"he wasn't that way at first."

"How do you mean?"

"It's funny how clearly I recall raising Casey. I don't remember much about raising my first son, Reg. He's a civil engineer, you know, and doing real well for himself, though we don't see him much." Her voice trailed off with her thoughts.

"Anyway, as I was saying, I sure remember Casey. Maybe it's because Slim was there when Casey was born."

"Really?" the doctor was surprised.

Ethel nodded. "Mind you, in those days, most men avoided delivery like it was the flu. But not Slim. He'd missed out on Reg's birth because he was working as a game warden at the time and was off near the Idaho border. But he said he was going to be right there beside me this time, just to make sure

Fannie, that's my sister, didn't try to slip in twins on us. You see, Fannie and Hazel Two-dog, she was a Blackfoot woman from over the pass, had offered to help with the delivery."

"How did they feel about your husband being there?"

"Hazel Two-dog didn't care. The more the merrier was her feeling. But Fannie almost had a conniption fit. 'I never heard of such a thing.' She began to fuss. 'He'll just be in the way and for no good purpose.'

" 'Well, hear it now,' I told her firm. 'Slim was there for the making of the baby, and if he wants to be around for its delivery, I guess that's his right, too.' Fannie didn't say another word. Of course I knew that talk about making babies generally left her flustered and speechless, anyway." Ethel laughed.

"Still, Fannie stewed about it for a long time. In fact, Slim said Fannie was so peeved when my time came and he went to get her in the sleigh that she sat on the back end, as far from Slim as she could get. I guess Hazel Two-dog rode in the seat next to him. Unfortunately, what with her being so fat and all, and Fannie way in the back, the sleigh rode heavy on the snow, and that's probably why it broke through the creek ice."

"So you were delivering at home?"

"In a warden's cabin out on Fast Creek," Ethel said. "You know, it's odd the things I remember. Like the flattened coffee tin covering a knothole in the ceiling above our bed. Hills Brothers Coffee, red and white lettering, with a picture of these three wise men in robes and beards. One was carrying a cup like he was taking it to the Christ child." Ethel stopped momentarily, considering the memory. "I'm Mormon, so of course I was wondering why wise men would be taking *coffee*, of all things, to the baby Jesus. Then I got to wondering how we came by that can in the first place." She smiled. "Course I knew that it was Slim's doing, probably put that particular can right there just to get my goat." Her smile grew into a grin.

"Anyway, I lay there just staring up at the ceiling, but still only vaguely present in the lull between the pains. Mind you, I wasn't feeling particularly anxious, but I do recall hoping that Slim would be there for the delivery. I hadn't any problems with Reg, and I didn't expect any with this one. Still, when the spasms started coming closer together, I will say that Casey's labour caught me pretty hard. I guess my water must have broke because my legs and the sheets were suddenly soaked, and I remember a feeling of embarrassment, like I'd peed myself in public. But that didn't last long because I realized the baby was on its way, and there wasn't any way of stopping the process. Still, you know, I wasn't scared. Maybe by then I was acting on instinct, holding my knees, spreading them when it felt right. The baby began to move as I pushed until suddenly a blinding pain shot through me and I almost went unconscious. I knew something was terribly wrong. I could feel with my fingers that the top of the baby's head was partway out, but it would come only come so far, and just as soon as I stopped pushing, it pulled back again. I guess maybe that's when I lost control." She set down the empty teacup and looked directly at the doctor.

"Slim said he could hear me screaming two hundred yards down the trail. The sleigh had broken through the ice on the creek and they'd had to walk the last quarter mile. Slim said he near died of fright when he ran through the door, what with me screaming and the bed soaked with blood and all. Course I don't recall any of it. I kinda remember grabbing his hands, though. And I must have dug my nails pretty deep into them, but he didn't say anything. In fact, Slim just started talking to me with that gentle southern Mississippi accent of his. I couldn't for the life of me tell you what he said, but I could feel his calm sweeping over me like a warm breeze."

"What was the problem?" the doctor asked.

"Well, Fannie told me later that the cord was wrapped around the baby's neck and shoulders, and when the head came partway out, the cord would pull it back in as soon as I stopped pushing. Hazel Two-dog, God bless her soul, saw right away what was happening, and when my pains eased a bit, she moved the baby back and brought the cord over his head. And of course, that was that, and the next time the spasms came, the baby passed without any problems at all."

The doctor sat, staring transfixed at Ethel. "I've never had children, I can only imagine what it's like."

"Well, I've often thought about that moment and I still can't explain it." Ethel paused. "I've never felt so close to death, and yet I've never felt so close to life, and somehow they didn't seem that different!" Ethel said it as much to herself as the doctor. "I recall hearing a high hee, hee, kind of a laugh like two poplars rubbing against each other in a wind. And I think Slim must have said 'Oh, my Gawd!' about a hundred times. Then I heard the baby's cry! Oh, my, that was a wonderful sound—the first cry of my baby. But then in that same one glorious moment, something very odd happened—something I don't really understand." Ethel hesitated. "It was as though I passed through a curtain. Everything was so silent. There was no sound, no cabin, not even the baby. I was somehow detached from the world of humans, of pain and joy. And suddenly I felt engulfed by light. No, that isn't quite right, I *was* the light, pure white light, energy, heat, maybe even life itself!" Her eyes sparked with excitement.

"But then something even stranger happened. For just as I was letting go and I could feel this warm comforter drawing me into sleep, I was all at once caught by a feeling even more powerful, even more primary. Part of me wanted so badly to give in to the light, but I couldn't, not without my baby. He was still attached to me even though they'd cut the cord." Ethel stopped for a moment, her words stirring up another thought.

"I guess you never really lose that feeling, the feeling that they're still attached. Somehow they're still part of your body, even when they're grown." She looked at the doctor. "I wouldn't have a baby like modern women do, with drugs and all. I don't believe you can understand the fullness of a mother's hold until you go through the whole process. But I'll tell you for sure, cutting the umbilical cord doesn't sever the child from its mother. Maybe that's why I never gave up on Casey: he's still attached."

The two women sat silently looking at the coffee table before them.

Ethel smiled finally. "You should've seen Slim when he brought Casey to me. You'd have thought he was carrying a fine piece of Montgomery Ward crystal. I can still picture his eyes. So proud and full of tears.

" 'Looks just like me,' Slim crowed, grinning at the baby,

'wrinkled like a parched prune!' Course, Casey does look just like Slim, same eyes, same nose—though Slim's has been broken some. Still, you can't mistake whose son that boy is. Even now, twenty-five years later, they're dead ringers for each other, both of them long and thin like shotgun barrels. And you know," she said earnestly, "when I saw that man holding his child, I wanted nothing more for that baby than to be just like Slim!

"I recall that night, as Slim and I lay on the bed with Casey between us, just talking into the night the way we do sometimes. We both marvelled how that little thing could one minute be a piece of you, like a leg or an arm, and then the next minute, it's a person. A person already with some instincts to fend on his own. Like the moment Slim laid Casey on my breast, and that tiny little mouth began suckling, just like he knew all along what he was supposed to do. It was then, as we lay there, that I told Slim about the feelings I'd had when Casey was born, about the light and all. I knew he'd understand, and he did. 'Ain't never been so close to the hand of God myself,' he said."

Ethel stopped. Her back was beginning to hurt from sitting so long. She stood and, placing her hands on her hips, she stretched slightly and walked to the window.

"What can you tell me about Casey's childhood?"

"Well..." Ethel returned to the couch and stood for a moment before sitting down. "I don't remember him being a particularly difficult baby. His older brother, Reg, found him hard to handle, but I think that's because Casey wouldn't take any of his bossing. I did have to laugh once, though. I'd gone over to the Rigbys to deliver some huckleberry preserves and I'd left Reg to give Casey a bath. Dead of winter and cold as a railroad spike. Well, when I come home, there was Casey jaybird naked out in the snow, and yelling like a cavalry officer at Reg. And Reg was standing in his bare feet on the last step of the porch waving a hard scrub brush and just bawling for being so mad. You never heard the likes! Casey didn't know many swear words back then—he wasn't but five or six at the time—so he was catching Reg's curses and flinging them back at him like snowballs. I finally had to put an end to it when

Casey started throwing hard chunks of ice at Reg." Ethel laughed. "Reg and Casey never have gotten along, but Lord, don't ever come between them. Then you'd think they was Siamese twins!

"But really Casey wasn't bad, maybe a little mischievous, but never with any evil intention. He was just full of himself. So happy and fired up for any adventure that might turn a dollar's worth of excitement. Slim said the reason Casey acted like he was part Indian was because Hazel Two-dog delivered him. But the truth is, he wasn't any wilder than Slim himself. Spunk and vinegar—and, of course, a double dose of the mountains in him. Even now, Slim and Casey are like two sled dogs. The more worrisome the weather and the tougher the going, the better they like it."

"How did Casey lose his arm?" the doctor asked.

"A hunting accident," Ethel said, shifting her thoughts forward in time. "You know, doctor, it's strange. Slim says I make worrying a science, but twice now I've had these strong premonitions before something awful happened. Actually, they were more like visions. The first time was when my best friend's son was killed in an avalanche. When he and two of his buddies stopped by the ranch to deliver a message on their way over the pass, I knew something awful was going to happen. I pleaded with them not to go, but they were set on taking some girls to a dance in Idaho that night and couldn't be talked out of it." A sadness came into her face. "Well, when the main slide broke loose, you could hear it clear across the valley. I ran all the way into town in my house slippers to be with my friend when the news came.

"The second time I had a bad premonition was the day Casey went with his cousin Oliver on his rural mail run. I didn't want him to go and I told him so, but Casey thought I was protecting him too much. Slim was down at the ranch trapping mink and I knew how it grieved the boy to be cooped up during the winter without his pa around. So I finally gave in.

"As Oliver told it, he and Casey were taking some mail out to the village of Elk Horn, about fifteen miles north of Skyline. It was November, and I recall there was already a lot of snow on the ground. Well, as I understand it, Casey had Slim's twelve-gauge shotgun along, and this flock of geese lifted up out of Paul Elich's grain field. And of course, the boys figured they'd get a couple of birds for Thanksgiving. Casey downed one goose clean on the first shot, but he just winged another with the second barrel, and it landed crippled in the field farther up the road. I guess Casey reloaded the gun and stuck it butt first in the cab through the window, then jumped on the running board while they drove to where the wounded bird was.

"From what Oliver said, Casey reached in and grabbed the gun by the barrel. But it had fallen between the mailbags, so he took it with both hands and started to drag it out. Fortunately he was still on the running board and leaning back from the barrels. Oliver figured that the strings on the bags somehow hooked on the triggers...and both barrels went off!"

"Oh, my God!" The doctor gasped.

"Thank the Lord, Oliver kept his wits about him. Right away he made tourniquets out of strips of canvas from the bags, and then he went straight to the hospital. In those days, the hospital was just a log building next to the Episcopal church. Before the accident, Slim used to joke that the church and the hospital were close so just in case they couldn't cure you, they still had a chance to convert you before you went knocking on the Pearlies. Anyway"—she returned to her story—"we only had one doctor, Doc Duprae, for the whole region. Thank heavens he was home and not off on a house call, so by the time Betty Rigby fetched me up, he was already there."

Ethel returned to the couch and sat down, accepting the offer of more tea.

"The operating room was pretty makeshift, as I remember, with just a long table covered with a pad and a sheet, and another one, hardly more than a spruced-up kitchen table, holding the surgical tools. They did have two bright reflector lights that washed everything in a kind of waxy sheen like that imitation fruit some people put up for show on their sideboards. A nurse tried to hold me back at the door, but I told her straight out that my son was in there, and she wasn't strong enough to keep me out.

"I walked right up to the table. Dr. Duprae was just cutting off the remnants of Casey's wool coat and shirt. Oh, Lord." She shuddered. "When I saw my boy, I just shook with sickness. He looked so small and frightened, like a rabbit that had been savaged by dogs.

"*Both* arms had been shot! The right one was almost completely gone. There wasn't any elbow left, and what remained of the muscles around it was shredded like gutshot meat." Her voice faltered. "Casey's left arm was a mess, too. The doctor said the bone was broken in at least a half-dozen places between the wrist and the elbow, and the skin was black and shiny from powder burns. Everything was soaked with blood, in spite of the tourniquets Oliver made, but believe it or not, Casey was still conscious! Oliver said that he never once passed out! Can you imagine?

"Well, when Casey saw me, the tears just flooded from his terrified little eyes. 'Look what I've done, Mama.' His voice was faint and came in gasps, and it scared me to the core because I could hear how little strength he had left.

" 'Is it bad, Mama?' he asked, desperate to know the truth.

"I wanted to tell him different, but I just couldn't lie to him. 'Yes, son, it's real bad.'

"His eyes darted across my face. 'Am I going to die?' he asked.

"My breath came hard and I felt like I was choking, and for a minute nothing came out. 'No . . . no, son, you're not going to die,' I said finally, '*that* I am sure of!' I said it maybe as much for me as for Casey. 'I won't let you! We're gonna go through this together.'

"The doctor studied the wounds, prodding and talking to himself. Then, while the nurse began cleaning Casey for surgery, he took me off in a corner of the room by the window. I remember the snow outside looked so clean and untrampled, and oh, how I wanted my life to be just like that snow. I wanted it all to be a bad dream. I wanted my boy to be whole again!

"Finally the doctor touched my arm. I'll never forget his

face—even now it's as vivid as a catalogue picture. How can I describe it? Tired. Bone tired. Like all the pain and suffering he'd seen in his life had finally welled up in his eyes.

"He took my hand. 'Is Slim around? You and him should make this decision together.' I told him Slim and Jep were out on the trap line."

"Jep?" the psychiatrist asked. "Who was he?"

"He's a Sioux gentleman that works for us there on the ranch," Ethel explained.

The woman nodded. "I'm sorry for interrupting. Please go on."

"Well, Dr. Duprae figured there wasn't enough time to get Slim. 'Ethel,' he said to me, 'in spite of the tourniquets, Casey's lost a lot of blood already, and if we wait much longer he'll go into shock. You saw for yourself, Casey's right arm has been completely severed, and the best I can do for it now is stop the bleeding and close off the stump.' Then he paused, picking his words, 'I've got to tell you outright that my first concern is for the boy's life. That's the critical job ahead of us.' Again I saw the pain in his eyes. 'What I'm saying is, I don't know how much I can do for the left arm, Ethel. It's my opinion that they'll *both* have to come off.' "

Ethel looked at the carpet. "Well, his words were knives through my heart. A twelve-year-old boy with no arms for the rest of his life!" she said without looking up.

"I guess the doctor thought I'd just accept what he said and go along with his advice, but I couldn't. 'Take the one,' I told him, 'but not both!' It surprised me, too. But as soon as I said it, I knew it was right.

" 'Ethel,' the doctor pleaded with me, 'the boy might die! Bringing everything together could take too much time, and like I said, shock from blood loss is a real danger.' But I could see there was something else working in his face. Finally he came out with it. 'Even if Casey lives through the surgery, I doubt the left arm will ever be usable! Ethel,' he said, 'I'm just a country doctor, I'm not a surgeon!' His silence begged me to change my mind.

" 'Not both!' I said, firm. 'My son may have to be crippled for the rest of his days, but I won't make him an invalid!' I knew full well what I was asking of the man. Still, I couldn't do otherwise. 'Just do your best, I'm not asking for any more than that,' I said, looking out the window at the snow. I couldn't wish for things to be different, I knew what was ahead. 'I'll keep Casey alive, don't worry.'

"The doctor scrubbed in a metal basin and had me do the same. Then the nurse gave us both gowns and I sat down on a high stool near Casey's head. Casey and I have the same blood type, so they taped a thin transfusion tube to my arm and ran it down along the edge of the table to a needle taped to Casey's left leg. I remember looking at the apparatus that fed gas into Casey's mask and noticed 'Orvus' written on the glass bottle. Aren't those the people that made Slim's fly rods, I wondered. Well, that was just enough of an opening for Slim to come flooding into my thoughts. But I caught myself." There was an edge to her words.

She straightened her back. "I just put my hands on Casey's forehead and started talking to him even though he was already asleep from the gas. Just talking. Talking like Slim done to me when Casey was born. I told him the family stories about how my ma and pa had come across the prairies in a wagon. About how Slim trailed cows north to Wyoming from the King Ranch in Texas. How he'd tied with a fellow for top prize in the Cheyenne rodeo. And how Slim kept the saddle and gave the money to the other guy because the man had a family and Slim was a bachelor at the time. I told him about Slim walking into that barn dance at Schofield's and just sweeping me away.

"But most of all, I told Casey that he wasn't going to die. I talked to him about all the things he'd do when he got better, the fishing and pack trips that we'd all take together." Ethel drew in a deep breath. "For five hours I held onto that boy's life while Dr. Duprae worked—and I felt every cut like it was my flesh beneath the knife, like it was *my* right arm wrapped in towels and lying in a pan on the floor under the table. But finally, when I thought I couldn't take any more, the doctor stopped cutting and sewing and began bandaging Casey. And when he was sure he'd stopped the bleeding, he took the tube from us."

"How did your husband find out about the accident?"

"Well, as soon as my other son heard that Casey'd shot himself, he took a team and sleigh down the canyon to the junction where the road branches into the ranch. From there he snowshoed the ten miles up the Palmer River to fetch Slim. Luckily, Slim and Jep were there at the ranch and not out at one of the line cabins. They got back just as Casey was being moved to the recovery room.

" 'Slim, I remember saying when he walked through the hospital door, 'you look like Methuselah.' It was a silly thing to say after all I'd been through; strange what comes to your mind when you're tired and fragile. But Slim *was* a sight, what with ice hanging from his hair and off that beard he'd grown out on the trap line. And the poor man was so exhausted with fright and from the trip out.

"I pulled my strength together and told him all of it, the accident, the decision to try to save the left arm. He listened to me clear through to the end and he didn't say a word. And for a long time he just stood there in the middle of the room, looking at the puddle of melting snow dripping off his leggings and pooling around his packs.

" 'You done the right thing,' he said finally, his jaw set hard. 'One arm, no matter how twisted, is a far sight better than none! And Casey's a fighter, he ain't gonna let it hold him back.' His voice was so full and reassuring that it carried away my last reserves, and I cried in his arms for a long, long time. I cried for my poor mutilated boy and for me and what I'd lost. And I guess"—Ethel cupped her hands together in her lap—"I even cried some for Slim, because I knew he'd never do it for himself."

The doctor reached over to lay her hand on Ethel's.

"When I was empty," Ethel said, straightening her back once more, "Slim took me over to a bench in the hall. 'Ethel,' he said, 'whatever happens with Casey's remaining arm— whether he gets to use it again, or whether it eventually has to come off—we ain't gonna raise him like a cripple!' Slim knelt in front of me, looking at me level. 'We ain't *never* going to treat him different than we would if he had two arms! Do you hear what I'm saying?' His eyes searched mine. 'You can't mother him whole! What's done is done and them's the facts we got to live with.'

"Oh, Lord, how it hurt me, because it sounded like Slim was asking me to stop a river that flows so free and natural from a mother. But I also understood that it had to be that way, and finally I agreed.

"Over the next few years that's the way it was. And I came to abide with so much pain and frustration, trying not to treat Casey like he was crippled. And there wasn't a day that passed when I didn't have to catch myself from swooping in and doing for him more than I did for Reg. I held back, but can you imagine my agony, watching that child as he had to relearn how to do even the simplest things like just moving his fingers. Sometimes he'd get so frustrated he'd scream for anger.

"His first task was making the arm work. Dr. Duprae had done a much better job than he'd admit, and the movement in Casey's fingers came along pretty fast. But the muscles around his wrist and elbow were badly withered. Looking back, I guess now it's kind of comical the way Casey built up the strength in his arm. When he got out of the hospital and back to attending school, he'd carry his books in a pail, up close to his body, because that's the way the doctor set the arm—folded across his chest and all.

"Well,"—Ethel laughed lightly—"Casey was determined to straighten out that arm come hell or high water, so he took to packing rocks in the pail, and he'd add a rock each day until finally he got the arm pulled straight. But of course, he couldn't get it to bend up again, and it hung by his side like a plank. Then one day he was roughhousing with some of his pals after school and, don't you know, Casey fell and his arm folded up again. Well! When he saw that the arm could be bent and straightened, he started right away building up the muscles. In fact, now, if you notice, Casey's arm is as big as a leg of lamb and his hand is the size of a baseball mitt. Guess that's why he was so good at rodeo." Ethel smiled proudly.

"Holding and pulling things was a big problem for him. And there wasn't anything that came as hard for him as learning to tie his shoes. He could get his fingers to make the slip knot but he couldn't draw the bow tight for love or money. He'd get down on the floor with his foot pulled under him, trying to use anything from his teeth to his stump for help. I'd watch from the kitchen, just aching inside to help him. But he finally did it. He figured out he could pin half of the bow with his other foot against the side of his shoe so his fingers could work on the knot until he got it right. After some practice, he got it perfected, and I sure had to laugh when he tied together every one of Reg's shoes in the closet. And don't you know, there was some fussing over that!" Again she laughed.

"He never looked back from then on. And I'll tell you for a fact, there isn't anything he can't do with that one arm. And a lot of things he does better than most men with two. For example, he's a crack shot with a rifle. Slim says he can shoot the flame off a candle without touching the wick. But it's true. He'll sling that rifle of his across his stump." She raised her left arm as though it were a rifle rest, and with the other hand she seemed to grip the stock and trigger guard. "And without a flinch or a flicker, he'll put a bullet right where he wants it every time." She squeezed her index finger.

"No fooling. There isn't a thing Casey can't do. The boy's got gumption when he wants something." Ethel smiled. "But I will admit, he sure has an odd way of *not* showing it sometimes. Like the deal with the ski jumping and the rifle." She stared at her teacup as though reading the leaves. "You see, Olas Johnston, the Olympic ski jumper, moved to Skyline with his brother, and the two of them talked the ski hill people into building a jump, for training and teaching and all. Well, there was always a passel of kids hanging around it, and I guess Casey must have been one of them because one day Olas came up to me in front of the post office and asked if it would be all right to teach Casey how to jump. I worried about it some but Slim thought Casey needed something to spark his fire that winter, so we agreed to let the boy try. Course, for the next few weeks after that, ski jumping and telemark landings were all we heard around the house.

"Then, about that time, the *Statesman* newspaper decided to sponsor a junior jumping contest, and they put up a beautiful 25-35 rifle for first prize. Well, you wouldn't believe the activity that hubbubbed around the jump! Kids were out there like a bunch of otter pups, up and down, up and down from sunrise to dusk. Everybody was practising for that rifle. Everybody, that is, except Casey! No sooner had they announced the competition than he *stopped* hanging out at the jump hill.

"The contest was the biggest event of the winter. The whole town showed up, and lots of families came in from the surrounding ranches. Even Hazel Two-dog and her whole clan came over the pass, hoping to watch Casey. I noticed that Casey brought his skis with him, but he was so casual that you would have supposed he was there just for the free popcorn.

"As I recall, Slim and I were standing with Olas near the run out of the hill, and he was encouraging each boy. 'Nice jump' and 'good improvement,' he'd tell them when they'd finished. When pretty well everyone had had their chance, the announcer asked on the loud-speaker if anyone else would like to try. That's when Casey, way up on the intake ramp, waved his good arm. 'Watch this,' Olas said to us as Casey came down the approach. Well! When he snapped off that jump, it was the most beautiful sight you've ever seen. He just hung there suspended in the air, soaring like a magnificent eagle. Out over his ski tips with his arm pinned against his side, his eyes fixed on the horizon. And all you could hear was the wind flapping through his wool britches. It was as if everyone was holding their breath.

"But, when he landed and dropped into that telemark, boy-howdy, the whole hill was yelling and cheering for him. And don't you know, he set the jump's junior record! Course, Slim and I had no idea he was that good.

"Olas told us that Casey was practising at night! He and Reg would sneak over to the jump after supper, and Reg would hold a lantern on the lip so Casey could see where to leap from, and Olas would stand with another lantern farther down the landing. Olas said Casey was a natural, and that he could be a world competitor if he had a mind to. But I don't think Casey was set on anything more than that rifle." Ethel stopped talking, following another train that intersected her thoughts.

"The rifle reminds me of something I've thought a lot about

lately." Ethel's eyes grew uncertain. "It happened when we horse packed some guests from the ranch into Yellowstone Park. In fact, it was John and Helen Mayfield and their son, Shag. We all called him that because of his wild hair. The Mayfields were our first guests, and they haven't missed a season since. Shag is Casey's age, and I think they were about fifteen at the time of the Yellowstone trip. That's right, because Casey had just won the 25-35 the winter before.

"Anyway, one evening we'd camped on the edge of a large meadow that was pocked with steam vents and grottoes and those hot mud pots and the likes. The boys went off exploring, and I guess what happened was, Casey got to showing off for Shag around one of the steam vents, and don't you know, he slipped on the slick mud. With only one arm and all, he had to throw the rifle to catch himself, and the gun slid back along a side wall sloping into the pit. Well, darned if those pups didn't decide to scramble in after it. And then they couldn't get out! And what with all the noise and steam hissing from the grotto below them, nobody could hear them calling either."

"My gosh!" the doctor exclaimed. "How on earth did you find them?"

"Well, fortunately, it wasn't very long before we got to missing the boys. And we began searching around the grottoes and geyser holes first, and it was maybe fifteen minutes later that we found them. Slim had to rappel down on a lash rope, and, boy-howdy, I'll tell you, we were all pretty frightened staring into that stinking steam and not seeing much of anything. When we hauled them up to the surface, those boys were choking and retching, and red, my Lord, they looked like two cooked lobsters. But, you know, Casey had his rifle!" Ethel shook her head.

"I could see Casey was really scared. So after all the fuss died down, I took him off alone for a walk. And when we got to a place near a pine stand where no one could see us, I put my arms around him and he started sobbing like the world was gonna end.

" 'Shag won't be allowed to play with me any more, will he?' Casey said finally.

" 'Of course he will! Why wouldn't he?' I asked him.

"He didn't say anything for a long while, then he blurted out, 'Never would have happened, Mama, if I'd had two arms!' And he started to tremble. 'Just before Dad reached us, I felt Shag starting to slip, and I had a firm hold of a ledge with my arm, but I didn't have another arm to reach out to him. Mama, Shag could have died and I couldn't have done a single thing to save him!' He began to sob again. 'Hell, Mama, I ain't no use to myself, or anybody else when it comes down to it!'

"Oh, Lord! If only I could have that moment to live over again!" Ethel looked sadly at the doctor. "But I just shushed him up cold. 'You're not a cripple!' I told him. 'Don't start thinking that way, because nobody else does.' It was what I always said when Casey had any doubts or self-pity, or if he came to me for sympathy. I guess somehow I thought that those ideas would just go away if they weren't given voice.... Out'a sight out'a mind. Now," she said, turning to the window and the light snow flurry that had begun to fall outside, "after all that's happened, I see now that those ideas *didn't* go away. I just drove Casey's feelings underground, back into that awful pit."

"What did he say then?" the psychiatrist asked, sensing the importance of the story.

"At first he didn't say anything, then he suddenly snapped back at me, 'Mama! I *am* a cripple, and damn it, I'm tired of everybody lying to me!' he said. Then he waved his stump in front of my face. 'Do you think I'm blind, too? I'm missing an arm, Mama! I don't have an arm!'

"Oh, Doctor," Ethel sighed. "There's so much I should have said, back then when he might have heard me. But you know what I did? Nothing! As usual, I held back, trying not to mother him whole." Ethel's voice was heavy. "And that was the last time Casey ever came to me for sympathy." She looked for some time at the window. Snowflakes were melting against the warm windowpane.

"In hindsight, I see he began to change after that, began turning inward. He became kind of single tracked, and real competitive. Mind you, he'd always given his all, but not to the exclusion of everything and everybody else. Take his rodeoing, for example. He was a real good saddle-bronc rider because his arm was so strong and powerful and all. But, you know, he wasn't like the other cowboys. Never hung around the grounds with them, either before or after the rodeo. He'd just show up and take his ride, then leave as soon as he collected what money he had coming.

"As it happened, Justin Fletcher, the rodeo stock promoter, took notice of Casey and encouraged him to try for the national finals at the Colosseum here in Denver. Well, boy-howdy, Casey worked. Every weekend he was in a rodeo somewhere, and according to Justin, he took top money most of the time. But that rodeo circuit is hard on a man, driving back and forth across the country, sleeping in your truck most of the time, hitting one rodeo, then on to the next before the dust settles from the last one. I worried that Casey was pushing himself too hard, but Slim said that's what it took to get to the nationals. Casey didn't talk much when he came home, not even to Slim. He didn't tell us how his rides went, like they weren't important to him. Most of the time, as soon as he got home, he'd take a saddle horse and a pack horse and disappear into the mountains for days on end until he had to leave for the next rodeo. Still, it paid off. He qualified for the nationals, and Lord knows we were sure proud of him.

"I can't rightly say what happened down here in Denver. First time we knew anything was wrong was when Justin called to say Casey hadn't shown up yet, but we just figured he'd wait until the last minute, like he always did. But when Justin called back to say Casey missed *both* his rides, we started to worry. Slim contacted the highway patrol, but they didn't know anything. Neither did the Denver police, or the hospitals, at the time. I was just beside myself. And we were fixin' to come down here to look for him.

"Then I got a call from my niece, Katie Haynes. Her speech was real slow and thick, and I could tell she'd been drinking. She said that Casey was in Denver with her, and that they were doing fine. Well, my heart just sank. Oh, I don't mean to bad mouth Katie. She was a fine little girl when she lived with us for that spell after her ma died. But the poor little thing always seemed to carry such a deep hollow place in her soul that we just couldn't fill. We loved her like she was our own, and she and Casey were the best of chums, which was good for both of them since neither of them had any close friends. Reg would rather have scalped them than befriend them.

"Unfortunately, after a couple of years, her father wanted her back. She wrote to us some, then the letters stopped. I heard later she kind of went wild there at Amos's and finally ran away with a saddle tramp. Can't really say I blame her much, out in that desolate prairie and all alone except for Amos, and he never was right in the head. You could tell. When he got on a pet topic like cougars killing his sheep, or damnation and salvation, you could see white all the way around his eyes. Slim said he'd been nursing on the wind too long.

"No," Ethel said with a sigh, "what set me back about Katie was that she was a down-in-the-gutter drunk. Also I'd heard from people who'd seen her in Denver that not only was she drinking hard, but she was selling herself on Larimer Street. Anyway, in the background I could hear Casey. He was yelling . . ." She drew in her breath, then released it. "Screaming just the most awful things about Slim and me. Calling us hateful names . . . and accusing us of terrible things." Ethel winced. "That's when he said it. He was sobbing, but I could still hear him clear. He said that there was one thing we gave Reg but never him, and you know what he said that was?" She looked reluctantly at the doctor. "Sympathy," she whispered with some difficulty. "That's what he said, sympathy."

"Humph." The doctor stared at Ethel with astonishment.

"Lord, it sliced me just like Dr. Duprae's knife cut into Casey. I pleaded with Katie to put Casey on the phone, but he wouldn't talk to me. Then there was the sound of glass breaking, and the phone went dead."

The doctor nodded. "I know the rest," she said. "I was the one who admitted him when the police brought him in. I ordered his stomach pumped."

Ethel's eyes questioned hers.

"Amphetamines and alcohol," the doctor answered. "A bad combination."

Ethel fell silent, twisting a small handkerchief and looking at her hands, at the swollen, inflamed knuckles and the cracks that would never seal, no matter how much lotion she put on them at the end of each day.

Then she looked at the doctor with sharp, penetrating eyes. "Sometimes," Ethel said, "sometimes at night, when Slim is asleep and I stare up at the ceiling, alone, like I did just before Casey was born, I wonder if Slim and me really did the right thing. Treating him like everybody else, expecting him to do for himself all alone..."

It was a long time before she spoke again. "Maybe he just got tired of pretending," she whispered softly, "tired of proving that he has two arms, when every day of his life he sees that it just *isn't* true." She lifted her head and faced the doctor. "Maybe by denying that he *is* crippled, we've crippled him in another way."

Ethel's gaze wandered to the hospital window again. The snow had begun falling hard in big, silver-dollar-sized flakes, and once again the pure and untrodden white blanket called to her as it had the day of the accident. She stood and walked over to the window. Again she wished things could be different. But of course, that wasn't possible, she realized. The past was gone, and it wouldn't help to wish.

Ethel collected herself and walked to the couch. Standing erect before the doctor, she extended her hand. "I'll see my son now," she said, giving the doctor's hand a reassuring squeeze. "And don't you worry none, he's going to get better. I know it now."

KATIE HAYNES

"MIND IF I SIT BY THE WINDOW?" KATIE SMILED AT THE MIDDLE-aged man in the train seat as the City of Los Angeles lurched out of the Denver train station and headed north across the desert. She felt his eyes upon her as she moved in front of him and sat down. Out of habit, her hands fluttered over the fringed blouse, grooming the ruffles away from her cleavage. For a fleeting instant she considered hustling him. But she caught herself, realizing that she couldn't do that any more. Soon she'd be a rancher's wife. Turning away from the man, she discreetly tugged at her lavender Levis, which had pulled taut into her crotch. With the attention she supposed a rancher's wife would take with an expensive coat, she removed her rabbit-skin jacket. She then lifted her powder-blue cowboy hat from her head, careful not to disturb her wig.

Although Katie's frame was slight, with a lingering hint of a not-so-distant youthful beauty, there was also a hardness only partially masked by rouge and eye liner. Her mouth was small and refined, but the heavy gloss lipstick made it look thick and garish. Her eyes, bedroom eyes, pouted languidly at the edges like the drooping branches of the river willow. Yet, deep in their hazel recesses, they receded like the two long train tracks reflected in the window.

"I come from these parts," she said finally, two hours out of Denver towards Green River Station in Wyoming. "Came from the foothills of those mountains." She pointed to the west, to a distant blue range, the first legions of the Rockies lifting out of a desert of sagebrush and sand dunes. "Going back, you know, to get married. A rancher, real nice guy, big place, too. We owned a *big* ranch when I was a kid. Lots of land and cattle and horses. I had my own horse." Her words rushed from her like bats from a sealed cave. "A real pretty thing, a palomino. Used to go riding all the time with Juanita, the cook's daughter. Oh, yeah, my ma had a cook! And a real big house! Pa had lots of men to look after the place and the animals. He took me everywhere with him, San Francisco, New Orleans.

"School? Weren't no school nearby. For a while I spent my winters with my uncle Slim and aunt Ethel and my cousins, Casey and Reg, and went to school there in Skyline. They was real good to me, Uncle Slim and Aunt Ethel—real good. She used to read me bedtime stories and he'd take me fishing—even being a girl and all. He treated me just like he treated Casey and Reg. Casey and I were best friends...." Her voice trailed behind her thoughts. "I kinda figured I'd maybe marry him someday, but then Ma died."

Katie had told the story so many times she sometimes wondered what was really true. She had lived a few winters with her aunt and uncle before her mother died, and she felt sure that they *had* loved her. And it was true that she was going to Green River Station to be married to a sheep rancher. But she knew, when she chose to remember, that her family had never had cattle, nor a cook, nor a big house, and she'd only seen pictures of San Francisco and New Orleans.

Still, she wanted to believe these things. Desperately, she wanted something other than memories of a clapboard and sod herder's shack on the wind-cut plains east of the Rockies. She hated her past, the only daughter of a sheepherder turned zealot come Sunday and a mother who shuffled silently through her featureless life, fearing both God and her husband, Amos, with equal apprehension since both could unleash their fury without provocation or warning.

Katie's mother died silently and inconspicuously from a small wire cut, which Amos had poulticed with sheep shit until finally the infection spread through her system too far for the doctor to stop it. Katie was ten at the time and left to survive on Amos's diet of sage, sheep meat and salvation. Sin, like the fine sand that penetrated every crack of the Haynes's cabin, was daily collected and weekly dispelled at the Sunday-night prayer meetings.

Suddenly, a hostile memory seized Katie as she looked out the train window.

"The sheep man is the son of Job!" the Reverend Jones bellowed, trying to meet the howl of the wind with equal volume and passion. "Like Job, God is testing your every fibre. I see it in your faces. I hear it in your voices. Yes, believe me, my friends, I *know* the challenge God has set before you," he comforted them. "And I wonder to myself, How will you meet this test of faith? Will you be caught in the devil's power? Will he carry you down the wide road to eternal damnation? Or. . . . " The reverend let his voice slide softly to a whisper; his eyes swept his small flock. "Like Job, will you choose to walk the narrow and often perilous path to eternal paradise? Will you say to Satan, 'Devil!' " —his voice rose— " 'get thee behind me!' " Katie's small hands began to tremble.

"We are all sinners," the voice stated flatly. "Sinners!" The reverend began building like rolling thunder; his hand rose above the pulpit. "And as sure as I'm standing here before you tonight, the Day of Judgement is upon us! And God help the man, woman or child who has not found salvation from his sins!" The hand came down hard with a bang. "God help them!" he repeated, letting the walls and the wind echo the threat.

"But Hallelujah!" His voice suddenly rang out like that of a circus barker. "Through the wonderful mercy of Jesus Christ, there *is* salvation! And when you're saved, you will, like Job, let suffering strengthen your faith, let hardship nourish your conviction. So I'm asking you tonight, as we sing hymn number 176, 'A Closer Walk with Thee,' to come forward, here in Christ's presence, and affirm your faith. Ask God tonight to accept you into His fold, to grant you blessed salvation from everlasting hell. Let us sing."

The congregation began a weak attempt to soften the wind's moan. Katie felt ill. She was a sinner, for she held hate in her heart, but it was a sin she didn't want to give up.

"Brothers and sisters," intoned the reverend, just audible above the battle between Christians and the desert's wail, "take that closer walk with Him. Tonight in God's presence, quietly leave your seats and come forward to meet your heavenly father."

Katie mouthed the words of the song. Her terrified eyes darted to Amos's face. He was staring at her. She jerked to escape the grip of his glare, but she would not rise from the pew.

Katie felt anxious and thought about the flask in her purse. No. She caught herself. She was going back sober. As the train toiled across the Great Continental Divide Basin, she focussed on the landscape beyond the window. Wandering sand dunes and wind sculptings off tumbleweed skeletons were signatures of the great windstorms that swept the basin, weeding out everything that wasn't anchored to the hardpan. Maybe that was her problem, she wasn't rooted deep enough before the wind caught her. Well, she resolved, it wouldn't catch her this time.

She hadn't thought about Amos in years, at least not openly, though all too often he came rudely into her dreams, dark and foreboding like an unlocked bedroom door. Suddenly her gaze fell upon the carcass of a dead antelope not far from the tracks. Maybe a train kill, more likely a winter kill. A straggler that somehow made it through the summer but gave up as the temperature began to plummet and the winds drove the cold like nails. She shuddered and looked away to the mountains. A snowstorm was building along the distant peaks. She wondered if Amos was still there. She hoped so. She wanted to see his face when she came riding back in a brand-new pickup, wearing fine Denver clothes, with Barry on her arm. He'd know then that she'd done good. For sure, he'd know then! She smiled.

"Green River Station," called the conductor.

Katie dried her eyes. Excusing herself, she made her way to the washroom in the back of the car. Her hands shook so, she had to hold the basin for a moment before taking the thin pint flask from her purse. She swallowed hard and waited for the first rush of fire before taking another pull. Finally straightening, she corrected her wig and studied her make-up. The eyes needed touching—always the eyes. She had trouble making a straight line with the eye liner, and finally she had to hold one hand with the other, to fill in where the tears had washed. She unfastened another snap on her blouse, but on second thought, she closed it. No need for that any more, she had her man.

The cars banged to a stop and still she didn't see Barry. What if he hadn't come? Her ticket was one-way. Then she spied him standing shyly in the shadows by the station door. His boots were shined, his shirt pressed and the hat in hand was new, with the factory curl still fresh. Suddenly, for the first time since Denver, she felt good about her decision to leave Larimer Street and come back to the east slope. Still, he looked much older than she remembered as he stepped into the sunlight. How would she look to him? Then, for a pulse, she saw something frightening in Barry's solitary face. His eyes were the eyes mirrored in the train window; they were her eyes—they were Amos's eyes. "The wind knows but one face," the Reverend Jones had said.

"Here I am!" she called from the platform. Barry waved. She could see the relief in his face, and again she felt reassured that she'd done the right thing. Still, she moved awkwardly towards him; after all, they'd known each other for only a few days in early October, and it was now mid-November.

"Here, I brought you something." Katie smiled, pushing a small package into Barry's hand. Inside he found a tooled gold disk, a concho from a saddle. "It's for your saddle horn, to remind you of me when you're out with the herd."

The concho stirred a memory Katie never wanted to forget. She got the concho when she was fifteen from a beautiful Shoshone boy. He came to the ranch with the cutting crew, mostly Indians and Mexicans who made a regular circuit of ranches in the spring to shear the sheep's winter fleece. He was young and undisciplined, with charcoal eyes ignited by a mischievous fire. His eyes soon found Katie, her hair grown long and feral like a horse's mane, her breasts full with prairie spring.

They traded looks in public and spoke circularly in private.

Fantasies disturbed Katie during the day as she watched him, half-naked, covered in sweat and lanolin, pinning the sheep between his legs with strong skilled hands.

And then one night, the last before the crew moved on, buried in a thick pile of sheep fleece, smelling of sage and lanolin, Katie let the young Shoshone enter her. He was her first man, though she'd explored herself with her fingers, sometimes painfully, imagining that's what a penis felt like. How different it felt holding the boy inside her. His movements were tender and gentle, not uncertain jerks and stabs. What pain there was passed soon, and she felt a growing hunger for him. She was a starving person given a banquet, and she never wanted to become full; she wanted to dine on his attention forever. But the sunrise came all too fast.

In the confused moments of parting, the boy self-consciously gave her the concho. He'd never held a white woman before without paying, he said, but his eyes betrayed that he loved her. And he promised to return at the end of the season to take her away, but he never came back.

"Full name and place of birth?" the court clerk asked Barry as he carefully filled in the marriage licence. Katie had changed into a pink cocktail dress and a small red hat with a white veil that she'd bought in a "new-to-you" store in Denver.

"Barry Cleveland Davis, Forty Mile Ranch, Kemmer, Wyoming."

The clerk turned to Katie.

"Katherine Alice Haynes, South Pass, Wyoming."

"Why, honey," Barry said, "that ain't but forty crow miles straight east of my place." Barry was astonished; he'd always assumed that she was a city woman, from Denver or maybe St. Louis.

"Oh, I was quite young when we moved."

"Age?"

Barry stammered. "Uh . . . fifty-two." The clerk entered it and glanced at Katie.

"Thirty-two, " she said without hesitation. The clerk's hand stopped before entering the numbers.

"Come on, honey, it don't make no difference how old you

really are," comforted the groom. He'd supposed she was in her early forties. "Tell the man your age."

"Damn it, Barry." Katie's eyes flashed with anger. "I *am!*"

"Oh." He scrambled. "I . . . I thought you were much younger."

"The judge will see you now. Please come this way."

Barry and Katie followed him to the door marked "Chambers." Katie glowed. She was really getting married. For all her fears, it was going to be good. She lowered the veil Ethel had sent her. Katie's mother had made the veil thirty years before. Katie wasn't sure why brides wore veils, but it was a tradition, and she wanted all the traditions there were. They seemed like armour against a best-forgotten past, backdrops for a new beginning. She stood erect and smiling beside Barry. Then she smelled it. Beneath Barry's heavy cologne, there was the unmistakable odour of mercaptan and sheep dip.

Mercaptan was the foul-smelling powder Amos stuffed in small pouches and tied around the neck of each sheep to ward off predators on the summer range. But in the spring of forty-four he missed one ewe he supposed still a lamb—Katie. And no sooner had Amos left with the flock for summer pasture than Katie fell prey to Ray Yoder, a saddle tramp who roamed those parts working the jobs (and women) vacated by men gone off to war or the munitions factories. That summer, dusk often settled upon Ray and Katie sprawled on the arroyo banks of the Sweetwater River, filling their needs to a chorus of meadowlarks and lovers' lies. It was a time of excitement for Katie. She felt deliciously sinful. But more than that, she felt the power of her body, for Ray was emotionally weak and physically aging and he desperately needed Katie's youth. She needed out. They would flee to the south, to the lights and sounds of Rock Springs, sheltered below the bluffs from the wind and the smell of sheep. Ray wanted to leave before Amos came back from the high country with the flock, but Katie wouldn't have it.

On the evening of Amos's return from the mountain pastures, Katie prepared a supper of sage grouse and beans. She cleared the table silently when the men finished their meal and rolled cigarettes. Then, in a flat, inconsequential voice, she said, "I'm pregnant." The lie had the anticipated effect: Amos lashed out, kicking the chair out from under the shocked cowboy. The Bull Durham sack flew from Ray's hand as he involuntarily shot backwards, his head crashing against the wood box. Amos threw the table out of his way and started for the stunned cowboy, but the deafening explosion of the shotgun resonating off the clapboard walls stopped him. Katie aimed the second barrel at Amos. Motioning Ray ahead of her, Katie moved towards the door, returning Amos's glare.

"Don't try it!" Her voice was clear and menacing. "You *killed* Ma and I should kill you for that!"

Amos's mouth twitched.

"Yeah, you did! You could haul me to town for those damn prayer meetings, but you couldn't bother to take Ma to the doctor till it was too late. Then treating her with animal shit." Her voice cracked. Amos shifted, but the violence flared again in Katie's eyes. "You murdered her, you bastard! Just as if you pulled a trigger. And that's one sin even God won't forgive! *Never!* No matter how hard you use me for barter!" Katie felt her strength weaken.

The race of the pickup's engine broke the spell. Katie ran outside, slamming the door and jamming a porch chair against it.

"Katherine! Come back here!" Amos bellowed .

Katie fired the second shot aimlessly at the side of the cabin and ran for the truck.

"Katherine!" The wood splintered as Amos threw himself against it. "Come back here!" he yelled, but the pickup was already moving down the road.

Two hours later, they pulled off into the desert, and with the radio blaring they made love. Wild and insane love that scared Ray, for long after he was spent, Katie clawed at his chest and shrieked at the night. Then, as the Sons of the Pioneers played full blast, she danced naked in the desert as though given to some invisible demon.

Katie and Ray drove into Rock Springs the following afternoon, moving into room 204 on the second floor of the Rawlins Hotel, Café and Bar. Katie grew bored with Ray when he drank, and the more fearsome Katie's wants, the more he drank, until soon "Ray the stud" became "Ray the gelding." But Katie wasn't content with one horse, and it wasn't long until she had a stable. "Wildly beautiful and beautifully wild," an admirer told her at her nineteenth birthday party. She was the queen of Rock Springs, and the Rawlins Hotel was her castle.

But Rock Springs was for miners, and Katie realized that coal dust eventually saturates the pores just like lanolin. She was ready to move. It was a rodeo cowboy, a saddle bronc rider from the circuit, who caught her fancy. Eugene was in the standings, which meant he'd won enough that season to ride in the championships in Denver. He was good, real good, and good-looking too—and headed for the city. The first day of the championships, Eugene drew a showy bronc, took top place in the bareback event and moved Katie into the Brown Palace Hotel, five stories higher than her room in the Rawlins and six and a half stories above Amos's sod hut.

"Our next contestant, coming out of chute number eight, is Eugene Robinson from Raton, New Mexico." The announcer's voice cut through the noise around the stock pens, building anticipation in the audience. They knew Eugene might win the all-round competition with this ride. Dancing from one foot to the other on the ramp behind the bucking chutes, Katie felt wild with the energy and tension. She gave him a fiery kiss, pressing her body to him as best she could. Eugene grinned to the gateman, proud of his woman. Then he settled onto the bronc and tightened his grip. For luck, he spat tobacco on the animal's mane. "Outside with this son of—" he barked at the gateman, but the words were lost to the explosion of the horse.

The first lunge beyond the gate drove Eugene hard against the horse's withers. The bronc cut to the right, throwing the cowboy far enough off balance that he had to drive himself backwards and claw with his spurs to regain his seat. But the rowels of his spurs missed the bronc's neck, and suddenly Eugene hung helpless upside down in the air, behind the horse. The bronc kicked at the top of its buck, catching the cowboy squarely in the head with both feet.

It had happened so fast. Katie stood frozen, not believing the motionless, distorted form in the sawdust was Eugene.

Cowboys poured from the chutes. A stretcher arrived and Eugene was carried to a waiting ambulance. As she got in with him, Katie saw that he was alive, but his hands felt cold and lifeless.

Confused, scared, Katie sat in the hospital waiting room until finally a doctor appeared. Eugene's spinal cord was crushed near the base of his skull; he'd likely be paralyzed for life. She felt paralyzed. She didn't know anyone in the city and she had no money, but she sure wasn't going home. Of course she felt sorry for Eugene, she told herself, but she hadn't bargained for life with a cripple, either. He was a trip to the city, nothing more. Katie stayed at the Brown Palace until the deposit on the room ran out, then she answered an ad for "evening work at Miss LaBane's Stockman's Club for Discriminating Gentlemen." Just until she got back on her feet.

The first years at the Stockman's Club were good to Katie. Her once lean fortune of a gold concho collected new friends as a rowdy stream of oil riggers and ranchers passed through her arms and legs. But Denver was becoming a suit-and-tie city, and business at the Stockman began to wane. Miss LaBane lowered her prices to stimulate interest, but the investments never came, only poorer cowhands, and not many of them. More and more, Katie found herself facing empty nights when no one came to hear her moans and feel her machinery. Her spring-ripe breasts began to sag like winter snowdrifts, and while the gin stopped the shaking hands, it also unlocked unwanted voices. More and more, Katie felt drawn from the Stockman to the aging bars along Larimer, catching an arm, any arm, laughing just for the noise to fill the night and mute the voices she heard when she was alone.

Then Casey arrived. God, how Katie wished he'd never come back into her life. He was no longer a boy, the best friend from those few wonderful years she'd known with Slim and Ethel; he was a man, like so many she'd come to know, hard and angry. He'd lost an arm in a hunting accident, and when he drank, which was most of the time, he cried for the missing arm and beat her with the remaining one. Still, for all the madness that surrounded Casey, she needed him, she told herself. Maybe if he sobered up, drew a good horse at the championships, they could both get away. Maybe they'd buy a small spread, start a family. But Casey didn't even get out of bed for the rodeo. He just lay there sick and crazy with pills and alcohol, until the police finally put him in an institution. She knew then it was over, all of it: the city, the dreams, even the precious memories of a distant innocence.

It was the day the *Denver Post*'s headlines announced, "Urban Renewal: A New Look for the Inner City," that Barry Davis walked into the Stockman. He'd come to town for a new saddle and "some honky-tonk times," but Katie made other plans and she gave him more than the usual fare, much more. She gave him tenderness and sympathy. Barry, his senses dulled by years of womanless solitude, basked in Katie's warmth, and within the week he proposed marriage and bought her passage on the City of Los Angeles to Green River Station.

The ceremony took less than twenty minutes. Katie and Barry emerged from the courthouse holding hands tightly.

"Well, we survived our first test, one more to go." Barry laughed.

As they crossed the street to the Rainbow Tavern, they were too happy to notice the light snow that began to fall. Or if they did notice, the fact was soon forgotten amongst the din of whoops and whistles that greeted them as they opened the tavern doors. Barry's friends hadn't waited for the bride and groom to start the party.

"Got yourself a looker, Barry," a fat cowboy congratulated him. "Course, ma'am," he said as he turned to Katie, "I can't say that *you* made much of a catch. Maybe you should throw 'im back and hook something better—like *me*, for example."

"The day it snows in hell is when this little lady's going to leave my side." Barry squeezed Katie's waist and accepted a drink.

Toasts were made to the couple. Fortified with hope and alcohol, normally shy ranch hands delivered sloppy advice on how to handle a wife. One old herder, his teeth gone from neglect, joked that a good beating was the key to keeping a woman. Brandishing her fist, Katie warned against it—much to the delight of the congregation. Katie was a success, and secretly Barry's friends were envious of his good fortune. More than one of them had lain awake at night, sick with the dread of dying alone. Barry had escaped; maybe they would, too. And Katie once again felt like a queen, this time with a king.

A large box cake had been bought at the bakery down the street. Someone had tried to scrape off the "Happy Birthday" with a pocketknife, leaving a blue swirl that looked to Katie like a child's finger-paint art. But she didn't care, it was a cake. It was tradition.

Outside, the sky grew leaden as night and the snowstorm settled in. Barry was anxious to get back to the ranch before the highway patrol closed the interstate. Besides, for a month he'd thought about this night. He'd hired the neighbour's wife to clean the house and make curtains, and he'd repaired fences and dragged derelict trucks and broken-down sheep wagons out of the yard.

Finally he rose to make the last toast. "May you all escape the hell of an empty bed!" He lifted and drained his glass. "And now," he added with a twisted grin, "it's time to git back to the ranch before this blizzard makes bed partners out of all of us." He raised his hand to calm the protest. "Me and my Mrs. got things to do and—" Katie blushed as the cowhands smiled at each other knowingly. "And I don't want to see any of your mutton faces sniffing around my back porch."

Thirty miles west of Green River, Barry turned his pickup off the interstate onto a rough gravel road. The light snow flurry was now a blizzard, but the truck cab was warm and Marty Robbins sang convincingly to them about hard times he'd shared with his "charmer darling." Katie could live with this man, she thought. She'd be proud of him, show him off to Amos.

Suddenly, though she was unsure why, for she couldn't see beyond the reach of the headlights into the snow, Katie realized she knew this stretch of road.

"Is there a church house around here?"

Barry nodded. "We just went past it."

Katie moved close to Barry, quietly absorbed in her

thoughts about coming back. Then, like an abandoned cat finally adopted, she rubbed against Barry's shoulder, kissing him on the cheek, playfully slipping her hand between his legs, watching him melt with her touch. Barry looked away from the road into his bride's face—just for an instant, but it was still too long. The truck jumped out of the rut. Barry cut the wheels back too sharp, and they skidded across the road, bounced over the edge of a shallow wash and crashed, still upright, onto the frozen desert floor. Katie and Barry rebounded off the roof, the contents of her purse emptying into the cab.

Katie was wedged between Barry and the steering wheel. The headlights on the driving snow created the illusion that the truck was still moving. Unconsciously Barry kept his foot mashed against the brake pedal.

"Oh, God, honey, I'm sorry! Are you all right?" He reached out to her.

She moved slowly back onto the seat. "Probably." Her head hurt, but she couldn't feel any blood as she ran her fingers through her hair.

Barry tried the engine. It started, but the truck bed sat at a strange angle. Still muttering how sorry he was, the sheepherder got out with a flashlight. It didn't take long to find the problem. When the truck hit, the right rear leaf spring had snapped, wedging the tire against the frame.

As he fought the door open against the wind, snow billowed in around him.

"Ain't too bad," he tried to assure Katie, "but I guess I'll have to go for help. There's a ranch house near here." He patted her hand then reached for the door latch. "It won't take long."

"Barry," Katie begged, "please don't go! Stay here and hold me till the storm passes." She wrapped her arms around his neck.

"That could take days. No, I'd better go now before the storm grows worse. But you'll be with me." Barry showed her the gold concho in his shirt pocket. He held her and they kissed with sincerity. Then, embarrassed with himself, he lunged against the door.

Barry disappeared so abruptly that his absence pulled around Katie like a vacuum. She sat motionless until the silence became intolerable. Turning on the dome light, she tried to discipline her shaking hands to pick up the contents of her purse. She was relieved to discover the flask, unbroken. Her eyes fell upon her mirror, broken. Taking the largest piece, she examined her face. The accident had thrown off her wig. Had Barry noticed? She found the hairpiece under the seat and quickly put it on and straightened it. Unscrewing the flask's cap, she drank from the bottle, then sat back, watching snowflakes imprinting vague images on the windshield. Again she drank, until the flask was empty. The alcohol comforted her. "The strength of Job." She laughed.

She dozed off, thinking about the wedding and Barry, but suddenly she was awakened.

"Katherine?" She heard something in the wind call out to her.

"Barry?" she asked, peering out the side window. But only the distorted shapes of driving snow appeared against the glass, growing more grotesque as her imagination raced.

"Barry won't be long," Katie warned aloud, seeking solace in the sound of her voice.

Silence followed her warning, and again she slipped into fitful sleep.

"Katherine!"

She bolted upright.

It was Amos's crushing bellow, the feel of bed sheets ripped away from a startled child. She shrank against the opposite door, pleading. She saw Amos's face pressed against the windshield, glaring at her.

"Katherine! Come here!"

"No!" she screamed. "Never! Never again!" She grabbed Barry's rifle from the rack behind her and waved it drunkenly at the apparition.

"Katherine!" wailed the wind.

The explosion shattered the windshield. The storm cascaded through the hole like water through a ruptured dam.

THE CLIMB

IT WAS A HEAVY PEWTER DAY AS THE LONE CLIMBER ASCENDED the alpine trail towards the cathedral of scoured peaks. Mud stuck to the soles of his climbing boots until he exploded with anger and gave each foot a violent kick, sending the clods sailing over the heather like startled ptarmigan.

Late October, and the mountains had already turned their faces towards winter—though not completely. It was a dangerous time to climb, neither fall nor winter. The snow fields were neither snow nor fields, but a ragged blanket of rocks and sedges braided together by thin snow skiffs. The unfrozen talus rock was still too loose for firm footing, and the lichen was soft and fish-skin slick. At least, he wouldn't have to contend with avalanches, Casey assured himself. Besides, he thought, if it were too easy, everybody would be doing it.

Oblivious to the driving sleet, Casey focussed on the trail. Though still in his early thirties, he walked hunched over as though burdened by age or by a heavy pack. He had grown a beard since leaving the hospital, but his eyes, sullen and intense, still betrayed a turbulent undercurrent. In one large, bare hand, he held an ice axe, which he used as a walking stick. There was no other hand, just a jacket sleeve folded over a stump and pinned back out of the way. His pack was a simple canvas rucksack on a wooden frame. But the coils of gold rope strapped to the top of it, and the belt of pitons and carabiners he wore around his waist, suggested that this was no casual climb.

It was not the weight of the pack that bent Casey like a snow-laden bough. In fact, his pack was light: a tent, a sleeping bag, a day's worth of food and water, a change of clothes and the climbing gear necessary for the assault. Casey knew every rock face he'd have to scale, every ice field he'd have to traverse. Twice before, he had attempted the climb. Both times he had been stopped short of the summit and the distinction of being the last climber to sign the peak's registry for the year. But this time Casey felt confident. He was physically strong, having trained all summer, and he was determined not to turn back, regardless of the toll.

Casey's burden that day was his thoughts. He had stopped at Sheila's cabin on his way out of Skyline early in the morning. He wasn't sure what she was to him. Girl friend? No, that implied possession, and no one possessed Sheila. Besides, if her ultimatum was to be believed, she was nothing to him now. Why in hell had she picked that morning of all mornings to start an argument?

They had never discussed settling down together, but Casey suspected that was the basis for her anger that morning, and he'd confronted her with it.

"I *wouldn't* marry you," she'd snapped at him, "not the way you are now."

"What do you mean, the way I am now?"

"You're obsessed with this climb. It's as if you're not here any more. You're already on that damn mountain. Lately, you look at people, but you don't see them. You listen, but you don't hear them."

"Better obsessed than useless." He'd laughed.

"You're useless now." She glared at him. "At least to everyone except yourself! There's no room for anyone else in your life. That's why Olas and the other guides won't climb with you any more—you're dangerous! Olas says you don't consider anyone else, that you go too far, take too many chances."

"So what do you want?" he'd retaliated. "Would you rather I became a porch monkey like Johnny Nisbett, sitting around at the mercantile talking about the things other people do?"

He remembered the infinite silence, interrupted only by the crackling of wood burning in Sheila's cook stove.

"Casey, I just want you to be a person. Forget that damn arm and stop trying to prove that it's still there!" She paused.

"Because, Casey"—she jabbed him with her finger—"if you don't give up this climb, my door will be closed if you return."

Casey hated ultimatums. He'd do what he damn well wanted, he grumbled as he stomped up the trail. She didn't understand the importance of the climb. And *he* knew why the guides didn't climb with him any more. Oh, they didn't say it outright, but to their thinking, a cripple was a liability. That's why he had to reach the summit, sign the registry, to show them he was *more* than their equal. And Sheila, she was just using the climb to manipulate him towards settling down with her—marriage, and babies, and the whole ball of twine. Casey's imagination raced. Maybe it was just security she had wanted all along. Why else would a beautiful woman like her settle for a one-armed man? In fact, maybe she thought that because he was a cripple, he'd be content to hang around her kitchen stove like a three-legged dog. Well, he assured himself, he'd given her his answer. And now that he was on the trail, he was glad of his decision. Again he gave each boot a sharp and violent kick.

His heavy mood slipped away as he climbed out of the last mutant patches of dwarfed fir and onto the scree slide. The slope became progressively steeper until finally he stood at the base of the first vertical head wall. He could see the chimney chute above the first face, and then the narrow horizontal ledge separating the chute from the second rock wall. The top of that face was shrouded in clouds, but Casey knew that above it was a long snow field leading to a climber's shelter. He would stay at the stone shelter that night and conquer the summit in the morning. October twenty-second. He smiled. Nobody had ever scaled the peak that late in the year.

He studied the surface of the first pitch, laying a mental route across the granite face, memorizing minuscule landmarks in case the clouds trapped him partway up. Then he unslung his pack and laid out a coil of rope at his feet. From the pack he took a small rock hammer and climbing harness. The harness, designed for him by Olas, was a simple hip-and-shoulder harness with a breastplate and a hook anchored at his chest with cross-strapping. It was his missing arm—his fourth point of contact with the mountain. The hook allowed

Casey to hang suspended either from his rope or directly from a piton, thus freeing his hand for setting new pitons above him. Because of his dependency on the harness, however, Casey had to use more pitons, at closer intervals, than a climber with two arms. It was a slow process, but at least he was climbing.

He stepped into the harness, adjusted the buckles on the chest plate and the crotch straps, and squatted a couple of times, making sure he could move his legs freely without being pinched or ruptured if he fell. Then he tied his ice axe to the back of his pack, carefully positioning the head so it wouldn't catch on his rope or, worse, impale him if he fell. Finally, he swung the pack frame onto his back.

Taking one end of the rope, he tied it with a bowline knot to his harness, leaving a long loose end for the prusik knot he'd tie to his down line. Then he began setting his first piton. The ring of the hammer driving the steel shank into the mountain echoed through him. He listened intently to each ring. If the piton didn't ring, but replied instead with a soft, hollow thump, it wasn't true and could give way just when he most depended upon it.

Like a spider laying the first tenuous thread, he moved steadily upwards across the face. Muscle control, mind control, self-control—balance and focus, the life-and-death facts of climbing, Casey often thought. It was the art of isometrics and motion. Of transferring tensions from one pressure point to another, clinging to slight hand holds and toe holds by sheer force. But change the angle ever so slightly, or relax the force a fraction, and the equilibrium was destroyed. It was the edge and the immediacy of the consequences that addicted Casey—self-control honed to precision by the penalty of a mistake. Climbing, he envisioned, was dance at its finest because one's very life depended upon the elegance of execution.

He worked his way up the face to the bottom of the chimney, a vertical crack in the cliff two feet wide at the base and spreading to more than three feet at times. It was roughly a hundred and twenty feet high. Again he removed his pack, but this time he laid it in the bottom of the chimney, positioning it so it could be easily lifted with a draw rope from above by a line tied to it. Then he wedged his hand and one foot against a wall and his back and other foot against the opposite side. Pressing himself between the faces with opposing forces, he inched upward like a caterpillar. Normally he could move faster, but the sleet left patches of black ice on the faces, forcing him to set pitons when normally he wouldn't bother. He considered setting a final safety anchor when he was thirty feet from the top of the chimney, but that would take too much time, Casey decided.

But, as he leaned forward to catch another pressure hold, the friction anchoring his right boot suddenly released. Instantly he was hurtled against the facing rock wall; then he dropped, free falling, helplessly slamming against the close walls on his way down.

Suddenly, Casey's body snapped as the safety line drew taut against the last piton and the ropes jerked the harness violently. He recoiled like a yo-yo a few feet up into the air before dropping again. Finally he hung, lifelessly suspended. With his arm and head drooping forward, he looked like a rag doll as he turned in slow concentric circles on the end of the line.

Casey convulsed to consciousness, his muscles suddenly twitching violently from shock and adrenaline. He gasped, but the pain in his ribs from the harness cut his breath to shallow gulps. His mouth tasted of vomit. Fright and pain confused his thoughts, and it took all his effort to gain his focus. Cautiously he wiggled his feet, then his arm. Nothing seemed broken. He folded forwards, then arched backwards, then forwards again, until the rhythm caused him to swing close enough to the wall to get a foot on it. He wedged back, and with his arm on the rope finally drew himself to the last piton, and hooked the harness into it. There he rested. Looking up, Casey saw that he had fallen only thirty feet. Finally collecting his strength, he again jammed himself into the chimney and began once more the slow caterpillar crawl upward.

His hands and feet were numb with cold as he pulled himself onto the narrow horizontal ledge at the top of the chimney. Though his heart continued to pound against his sore ribs, it was now a dull thunder. Exhausted, he drew his pack up the chute and collapsed onto it. But he knew he couldn't rest long, he'd lost too much time already.

The second wall was higher, but it had a slight back slope, making it easier than the first pitch and the chimney. Casey estimated he had at least two hours of daylight left; that would be enough. But soon the clouds descended, engulfing him, muffling the sound of his hammer. Time shrank to the needlepoint present and space to the cold granite inches from his face. It was only when his legs and arm began to cramp that he realized he'd been climbing for a very long time. He brought his watch near his face. An hour and a half had passed; he should have reached the top of the cliff. It must be just above him, he decided. But he found only featureless rock with fewer and fewer holds. A pulse of panic seized him—he was lost! He didn't want to descend, but what lay above? And he had to do something soon. The wind was beginning to build, increasing the chances of his being ripped from the wall by a gust and beaten against it like a hapless pendulum. Reluctantly he rappelled back to the ledge above the chimney.

It was getting too dark to try a different route or descend the chute. Casey realized he was stuck. He'd have to spend the night on the unprotected ledge and hope the weather changed by morning.

Taking his ice axe, he cut away the snow to make a level platform. There was barely enough room to pitch his tent. He drove a piton into the rock face behind and tied an anchor line from it to the peak of the tent. Crawling inside, he pushed his pack against the windward wall to break the force of the building gale, then unrolled his sleeping bag. But there wasn't enough room to lie down. He'd have to spend the night sitting with his back against the mountain. Too drained to care, Casey resigned himself to enduring the long night.

He sat there staring vaguely into the dark, listening to the wind scream around him, as he drifted between consciousness and dreams. "You've walked in somet'ing smelly t'is time," Jep would have said if he'd been there. Of course, Jep would never be there—he never did anything life-threatening just for the sake of doing it. Still, Jep didn't judge him. Slim and Ethel didn't judge, either, they just didn't understand him. At least, not since he'd been released from the hospital. Sheila understood, but she judged.

Casey's thoughts drifted to the evening he'd first met Sheila. It was at the Legion Christmas party. She was the new high school teacher and had just come to the valley from Oregon. He remembered watching her as she danced, her long auburn hair the tint of fall-red dogwood. He recalled how freely and uninhibitedly she'd moved, like a weightless dandelion seed swept back and forth in the breeze. He envied her laughter; it erupted so spontaneously. But it also embarrassed him, and though part of him longed to share her spontaneity, something cautioned him that it wasn't right.

"You shouldn't dance so!" He'd approached her between songs.

She shook the hair out of her face and stared at him with amusement. "Well," she said finally, "maybe you should!" She took his hand and hadn't let go.

That winter they went everywhere together, skiing, snowshoeing, ice fishing. In the summer they canoed on satin lakes while she flipped him with paddle water, on purpose, he supposed, since she would apologize profusely, then do it again. Though she teased him continually, he trusted her. In many ways, Sheila was like Slim and Ethel; she saw through people's pretensions. He'd never told her the details of the hospital, and pretended it was an experience of no consequence, but somehow she knew what it was like for him, insane and out of control. Yet despite her perceptiveness, she didn't seem to notice that he was crippled. Emotions came so naturally for Sheila; she laughed, she cried, she pinched and tickled, sobbed and hugged, screamed and moaned, cringed when she was frightened and threw things when she was mad. All he did was brag and swear.

She'd taught him to play. Except for the two short years when his cousin Katie had lived with his family, he had never played. What childhood there was had been wedged between chores and fights with his older brother, Reg. Then came the hunting accident, and there was no childhood after that. He was self-conscious at first because he didn't know the rules. With Sheila, however, there were no rules. She'd cheat at cards and bump the chess board when she was losing. She laughed when he was serious and tricked him when he least expected it. He didn't like that. Without rules, what was the purpose? "Fun is the purpose of fun," she'd argued. "Happiness is its own reward!" Anyway, Casey thought, getting married would have changed all that. Sheila would have had babies to play with.

Suddenly Casey lurched violently awake. The walls of the tent beat against his face. Then the floor beneath him began moving across the platform. The line to the anchor piton had snapped! Frantically he clawed at the floor, trying to dig into the snow, but with each gust the tent ballooned like a sail, dragging Casey towards the platform's edge. He released his grip and struggled frantically with his arm to find the door, but it was futile in the dark. Then his hand brushed the ice axe. Pushing its head up against the tent wall and the wind, he drove the shaft through the tent floor and deep into the snow below. With all his strength he pulled himself around the axe. Turning his back against the wind, he anchored the tent and it contents with his body.

"Please God!" he heard himself beg. "Not like this!" He was trapped. He didn't know where the door was, and he dared not move to find it. Again his fate was beyond his control, and he imagined the wind would somehow tear the whole snow ledge off the mountain's face. But it didn't, and eventually he saw he was safe as long as he hung on. Hooking his stump around the axe head, he reached down and drew his sleeping bag up around his shoulders.

"I've always figured dying alone wouldn't be so bad," Slim had once told him, "unless you're lonely, too." Casey had always been alone. He'd been close to death before; the hunting accident that took his arm, and once in Yellowstone when he'd slipped into a grotto vent. He was young then and somehow accepted his fate almost as an observer, but now it was different. Somehow Sheila had changed that. Against the mirror of death, he saw that he did not want to die alone. Also, if he survived, he didn't want to *live* alone, either!

Then it was over. He woke with a start. The wind had stopped. The tent lay exhausted on top of him. The thin, grey predawn light filtered through the tent wall, and the night of such indelible vividness suddenly became milky and murky. Slowly releasing his hold on the shaft of the axe, he painfully straightened out the muscles forged like steel bands into a fetal position. With his hand, he located the door and drew the opening over his head.

Suddenly he felt nauseated and dizzy. The storm had dragged the tent to the very lip of the platform! Just a breath beyond, the cliff fell for a thousand feet into a ravine of boulders and broken tree snags. If his tent had pulled just another twelve inches, he couldn't have stopped sliding. Already his pack, caught in the side wall of the tent, dangled freely out over the face.

Slowly he lay back against the ice axe and cautiously pulled himself towards the rock wall. Then, just as carefully, he drew the tent and his belongings to him, releasing a sigh of relief when he finally caught hold of his pack. For a long time he sat there, cradled against the stone wall with his knees under his chin, waiting for the first spike of dawn. The thin clouds far below were matted across the valley floor and looked like soft cotton gauze, white and sanitary. How different, Casey thought, from the dark and evil demons that just hours before had screamed around him, paralyzing him in their frenzy. All around him, blue peaks of ice and granite jutted out of the clouds like church spires and castle turrets above a mediaeval city. A magnificent, pristine citadel, he thought, and not of man's making.

As soon as the sun cleared the eastern horizon, Casey quickly drank the last of the water from his canteen and stuffed it, with his sleeping bag and the tattered tent, into the pack. His fingers fumbled awkwardly at the buckles on his harness. But no sooner had he moved onto the wall than he realized something was very wrong. His confidence was gone: he was scared. Fear diverted his attention, making him uncertain, and he moved with erratic jerks. Tasks that were once habitual had to be commanded by will. And twice he became so frozen to the wall by fear that he couldn't go on. Although eventually the catatonia passed, he made dangerous mistakes. Building a sling ladder, he tied a prusik knot backwards.

When he stepped into it, it slipped on itself, binding tightly around his boot, forcing him to free-hang from his harness to loosen the knot with his fingers.

Finally he reached the last piton placed the night before. As he looked up for a new hold, he was startled to discover that he'd turned back just a few yards from the top of the wall. Just ten minutes more, he realized, and the night on the ledge could have been avoided. Soon he cleared the edge of the wall, and within half an hour, he collapsed on the wooden-plank bunk in the climber's shelter.

Casey melted snow in his canteen over a candle and ate the last of his chocolate bars. Then he stripped his gear to just the ice crampons for his boots, a short safety rope and the axe he'd need for cutting steps in the last long ice shoulder leading to the summit. The rest of his equipment was stashed in a corner of the hut.

The brilliant sun off the vast snow field blinded Casey, and at times, when the ridge turned towards it, he had to squint through thin slits between his glove's fingers. Still, the sense of uncertainty that possessed him on the rock face earlier that morning melted away, and he felt strangely tranquil as he climbed. In fact, he seemed at times detached from the mountain, and he imagined himself as a bridge, linking the turquoise sky to the ivory crust beneath his feet. With mesmerized attention, he watched as his shadow raced across the snow ahead of him. It dove playfully into a deep indigo crevasse like an excited child in a game of hide-and-seek. He waved his arm for it to come back, but the shadow waved for him to come to the other side of the crevasse.

Removing the capstone from the summit's rock cairn, Casey reached down and extracted the tin canister and unscrewed its lid. There, rolled neatly into the tube, was the registry. As he opened the book, a gentle morning wind pulled at its leaves, stopping at the last page. Turning the canister upside down, he shook a short, stubby pencil out at his feet. He rested the open registry on his leg but did not pick up the pencil immediately.

Instead, Casey looked out, beyond the summit, to the vast panorama around him. It still looked like a great imperial palace, but the clouds had burned away, exposing a brilliant feudal tapestry of fall colours quilted together by green swaths of conifers. Far to the south, he could see thin trails of smoke from the stoves of Skyline. One would be Sheila's, he thought. Where before the valley had seemed barren and lifeless, it was now vibrant and alive. Still, though the majesty of the moment filled him with exhilaration, he did not feel exalted. He had reached the summit on October twenty-second, yet he felt only humble and very lucky. He picked up the pencil by his feet and stared for a long time at the registry. Then he lay the pencil in the book's seam, closed the registry around it and slid them into the canister.

Slowly he rose to his feet and looked for one last time at the world beneath him. He knew he would never return. Neither would he tell anyone about the climb. Sheila would know, of course. By his eyes, she would know every detail of the terrible night. Suddenly another realization crowded into his consciousness. Its force and obviousness surprised him, and he laughed. He would tell someone, he realized. He would tell Sheila and his children when they were old enough to understand.

CLOUD LAKE

CASEY GAZED AWAY FROM THE FRYING PAN, WATCHING A ROPE of juniper smoke as it curled out of the fire. It laced languidly over the carpet of moss to the platinum lake and the silhouette of the fisherman and his string of cutthroat trout. As the evening chill settled into the high alpine cirque, ghostly vapours rose behind the fisherman and twined around the shadowy horses grazing beyond. Primeval monsters emerging from an ancient lagoon, Casey thought. Great mastodons caught in an eclipse between day and night, life and death.

Suddenly Casey jumped as hot grease spat like a sparkler from the frying pan, burning the back of his hand. Cautiously he moved the skillet with the two slabs of trout away from the fire. As he did, his nostrils quickened to the smell of the frying fish blending with the lush, acrid scent of heather and edelweiss.

He listened as the mountain amphitheatre intensified the evening sounds. Even subtle whispers were given eloquent authority—a kingly command from the timid marmot or the cascade kettledrum roll from a single dislodged rock echoing through the peaks long after the mountain sheep had moved on to solid footing. Such brief melodies in the silence that held the cirque most of the year, Casey reflected. Brief celebrations of life wedged between ten months of deep snow and impenetrable winter.

Behind him he could hear the eider-soft lullaby Sheila sang to their son, her voice weaving easily into the tapestry of an alpine night. Casey, too, felt as if he'd emerged from a long winter of silence and Sheila was his spring. He smiled, remembering the day's events. Both Sheila and their son, Buddy, had caught their first fish that day. He recalled the laughing and shouting and the two of them running up and down the shore, their poor fish in tow, being inhumanely bashed across the rocks.

"She reminds me of Ethel," was the only comment Slim ever made about Sheila, but it was enough. And even though Sheila was rambunctious and impulsive, while Ethel was cautious, Casey knew what Slim had meant. Both women were gentle on the land. They moved easily with it, adjusting their step to its moods, bending effortlessly with its winds. It was understood that when Slim and Ethel retired, Casey and Sheila would continue with the ranch. And who knows, Casey speculated, maybe one day Buddy and a lady of his choosing would take over from them. And they, in turn, would guide fishermen to the primeval shores of Cloud Lake.

Shag Mayfield, Casey's client, approached the campfire with his catch, lake water still dripping from the fishes' tails. Although he had been coming to the ranch for years, this was his first trip to Cloud Lake. "Might not be paradise, but it's close enough for my money!" he said.

Casey laughed. "My sentiments exactly." Pointing with the spatula to the man's catch: "You've got a couple there that'll go four pounds, maybe five."

Mayfield smiled proudly, setting his rod against his tent. "I was wondering, down there by the lake, how in heaven's name did trout ever get way up here?"

Casey looked at the fire and didn't answer immediately. "Well," he said finally, "put away your fish and I'll tell you all about it."

The fisherman wrapped the trout in damp moss and laid them in his creel. After searching through the food panniers, he retrieved a bottle of Jack Daniel's bourbon and two tin cups.

"Oh, no, thanks, I've already got coffee." Casey held up his mug. "Besides, I'd never get through the story."

Shag sat down with his cup. "Well?"

"Well," Casey said, smiling, "there're two stories about these fish. There's the one I prefer to tell—and then there's the truth."

This amused Shag. "Start with the truth," he suggested.

"Naw," Casey said as though the matter was best dropped. "It's too unbelievable" He took a sip of coffee, savouring it, sucking in his cheeks as he swallowed, all the while baiting his friend.

"Tell you what," the fisherman rose to the hook, "give me *both* stories and I'll pick the more likely."

"Okay." Casey settled onto his haunches. "Now, the first theory is that the ancestors of these fish migrated here from Ptarmigan Lake, over that ridge." Casey pointed to a high rocky divide between two giant black peaks on the eastern skyline. "Now I haven't seen 'em do it myself, but tomorrow in the daylight, if you notice real close, there's some spaghetti-like lines running from that divide yonder, right down to the lake's edge. Some say they're trout troughs—migration trails."

Shag thought about this for a moment, apparently weighing the likelihood of trout scaling boulders and ledges for a thousand feet up one side of the mountain, then descending through equally rugged terrain to Cloud Lake. "That sounds to me like a shaggy fish story." He laughed, satisfied that nothing could be more absurd than the migration theory. "So, what's the truth?"

"The other story is simply that the trout were planted—if you can call it that. Probably strewn would be a better word—strewn and herded."

"Even that sounds more reasonable than fish climbing mountains."

"Humph." Casey chuckled. "I wouldn't be so quick to judge until you've heard the whole story. I'm not convinced—and I was there!"

Casey stared into the fire for a minute, then he began. "It all started with a band of mountain sheep. When I was a kid, back in the thirties, I heard a lot of guessing about whether or not there was a lake up here in this cirque. Nobody knew for sure, since nobody could find a way across that big rockslide, and that wall we came through today. But, then one fall when I was hunting elk near the base of the cliff, I spotted this band of sheep, mostly lambs and ewes, and one big ram with a set of horns about a curl and three-quarters.

"I didn't have a sheep licence, and besides I'm not much for trophy hunting, so I amused myself watching them through the glasses as they were walking at me across the slide, when all of a sudden . . . they vanished! Just up and disappeared, not a track or hair to be seen. Well, you can imagine my surprise. But soon I heard rocks clattering off a ledge way high above the slide, and I'll be damned if that ram wasn't standing on top of the wall!

"Course, right away I started looking around, and it wasn't long until I found their tracks going into that split in the cliff where we led the horses today. You know where I mean? Mind you, in those days the footing wasn't nearly as sound as it is now."

This amused Shag. "I'd say the highways crew could still do a little work on it. There were a couple of times there when I gave some serious thought to my loved ones back home."

"Good for you," Casey teased. "Makes you appreciate catching those trout.

"But, like I was saying," he continued, "I didn't see anything for a long time as I entered the cirque, and I was beginning to believe the whole basin was bone dry, when, wham! There she lay, clear and blue, like a satin sheet stretched taut across the bottom crater. God, what a sight! And so unexpected and all. I felt like I'd just discovered America." Casey beamed.

"The lake was so quiet and glassy that the clouds looked just like they'd fallen out of the sky and lay there beneath her surface. So I named her Cloud Lake. It wasn't very creative, but the name seems to fit, don't you think?"

Shag nodded. "Did she have fish in her then?"

"No." Casey shook his head. "But as soon as I got back to the ranch, I told Slim about her, and how I thought the lake was deep enough that she wouldn't freeze solid and just maybe could support fish. I figured the government hatchery people might supply fingerlings and we could pack them into the lake. Fisheries agreed, all right—provided one of their men, a guy named Millar, could come along. Course Dad wasn't keen on doing *anything* with fisheries. 'Ninety-day wonders,' was what Slim called government people, claiming they spent three summer months wandering around, wondering what the hell they were doing in the mountains, and then the rest of the year telling us, with their reports, just what they didn't discover. Still, Dad could tell it was important to me, so he agreed. But he warned them that it might get a little, as he says, owly! Which translates to being haywire to the point of turning outright dangerous.

"Since it was my idea, I remember getting up hours before the fisheries truck arrived, making sure everything was ready. Dad and I talked over breakfast about which horses were going and what kind of problems to expect. Like Snake Bait, he was this desert horse we'd got from the Shoshone, he wouldn't have his mountain feet yet so he'd have to be kept snubbed short and led along. And Whimples—she was my usual saddle horse—she'd have to be packed since she was one of the horses in our string strong enough to carry the dead weight of the fish cans up the mountain. Mind you, I was hard against it. Whimples, you see, was a fine, powerful horse, but she had a definite problem. She harboured a sadistic sense of humour. Like once, I remember, she carried me faithfully over two mountain ranges of tough elk hunting, and then, just a hundred feet from the corral, she started bucking like a rodeo bronc. Now, don't mistake me, I like the unexpected as much as the next fellow, keeps you young and alert—but not in pack horses! Unfortunately, Dad was still set to take her no matter what I said.

"Besides Millar the Wonder (as Dad called him) and Dad and me, Jep was coming along. I don't know that you know Jep," Casey said to Shag. The dude shook his head. "Well, he's a packer who's worked for the folks since before I was born. He usually doesn't come around until hunting season in the fall. I guess that's how you've missed him. Anyway, Jep is short for a Sioux nickname meaning eagle's crag, or so he claims. But it doesn't matter if the translation isn't exact, the name suits Jep to a tee. Every feature on his face has an angle to it: his brow, his nose, cheekbones, chin. And then his skin is stretched taut across them like leather on a drumhead.

"Judging only by Jep's eyes, people who don't know him usually think he's maybe a little mean—or maybe a lot crazy.

But the truth is, back then when we were doing the fish project, he was more kid than I was. In fact, that was the only fault my mother could find in him. 'Jep's a worker, I'll grant you that,' she'd say. 'And I don't know where this ranch would be without him,' she'd concede. 'But he ain't got a mason jar worth of ambition. He'll probably work for Slim for the rest of his life, and be happy to do it.'

"Well, that was just fine with me." Casey smiled. "And of course, Mom was always warning me not to get in too thick with Jep—so naturally we were as thick as thieves.

"But there was another reason I was glad Jep was coming along. He handles crises well. Ever notice how some folks just add more fuel to a crisis by getting excited? Not Jep, he never panics. In fact, there have been times when I *wished* he had more fire under his ass. Like the time he was teaching me to drive the hay truck and the front wheel's spindle shaft on his side sheared off.

" 'Tat's just wasteful,' Jep said, real casual like. 'Someone's t'rowing away a perfectly good tire.' (Of course there wasn't another soul around for forty miles in either direction.) 'Maybe we should stop. Could be our size!' " Casey began to laugh. "And naturally, because I was driving, I didn't see the rim and tire go bouncing down the embankment towards the river we'd been following. So I'm kinda wondering vaguely just what the hell he's going on about, and he just keeps on babbling away. 'We's gonna need one, tat's for sure.' he said, just about the time the front end suddenly augered down, and the steering wheel spun so fast that it rapped my knuckles about five times before I could pull back my hand." Absently Casey flexed and unflexed his hand. "I can still recall clear as can be the view in the side mirror as the three tons of hay tipped sideways in slow motion before they reached their balance point, then suddenly pitched over the bank to join the tire. Moose had a real feast that year."

Casey saw that the fish were ready. He stopped his story and shovelled the slabs of cutthroat onto three tin plates. "There's bannock in the Dutch oven, and pinto beans in the pot by your feet." Casey pointed with the spatula. "It's your own damn fault if you go hungry tonight." He was just getting ready to call Sheila when he saw her easing out of the tent so she wouldn't wake Buddy. She came over and joined Casey and Shag by the fire.

"Don't stop on my account," Sheila said as she sat down beside Casey, accepting a plate from him.

"Well, I was telling Shag about these fish." He pointed to her plate. "Anyway, the horses were all saddled and we'd finished our second cup of coffee when the tank truck finally boiled onto the ranch, blanketed in August dust. We were already late, and then, wouldn't you know it, the sound of the pump on the truck for emptying the fish panicked the pack string, and it took even more time to untangle them and sort out whose rope was strangling who. In the end, we finally had to take the horses out of earshot of the pump, fill each of the twelve containers on the ground and then bring one horse back at a time and pack him with a can on either side and lash them together with a barrel hitch. Jep was going to tie down the lids on the cans, but Millar said the fish's water had to be changed every four or five hours, so the lids were best left untied.

"I remember thinking, four or five hours! Hell, those fry would be swimming in Cloud Lake way before that. Dad was equally sure, and as we reined the pack string away from the hitching post, I recall him telling Mom to expect us back for supper. Fortunately, after years of living with Slim, she knew better than to expect us back before she actually saw us."

"A congenital disorder." Sheila nudged Casey with her foot.

Casey ignored her teasing. "At first, the cans rode well. But you could tell that the action of the water sloshing back and forth, plus the sun beating off the valley bottom, was wearing on the horses. And pretty soon every one of them was white with lather. In fact, I think they kinda anticipated cooling off at the Swift Creek crossing, because they sure picked up the pace as we got near to it. Now as you likely know, in the spring, Swift Creek can be a real nightmare, but by August it's no big deal—except, as you saw for yourself, in some places the water nozzles around those boulders with pretty fair force. Still, if a horse picks his footing and keeps his wits, there's generally no problem.

" 'Go on till you hit something,' was all Slim said to Trudy—you know, that big mare of his—and sure enough, she stepped off into the current without giving it a second thought. (Mind you, I think that horse would walk into hell if Dad asked her to.) I didn't have any trouble, either, bringing my string across, other than tears came to my eyes from the cold. But next was the Wonder, and he couldn't for love or money coax his horse across—mainly, I think, because he was pulling back on the reins instead of giving the horse its head. But whichever, they danced around the edge of the stream for quite a while, with him saying go, and signalling whoa.

" 'You still wants ta go with us?' Jep finally asked the Wonder, and I could see that the Indian was up to something. Wonder nodded in a maybe sort of way, but that was good enough for Jep. So, with the end of his lead rope, Jep gave the Wonder's horse a whack across the rump that you could hear clear across Swift Creek. God, the look on the Wonder's face! You'd have thought he was in the front car on a roller coaster. His eyes were closed so tight it was a miracle his whole face didn't break under the pressure. And the strangle hold he had on the saddle horn was so tight that he most likely left fingerprints in the leather!" Casey got to laughing so hard he had to set his plate down to keep from spilling it. Finally, he regained control. "But I guess there's a patron saint even for government men. When he finally came up on our side of the creek he was soaked like a piece of wet cowhide. But he was babbling happy just the same.

"Now that left just Jep on the other side, but he was leading Snake Bait, who'd probably never seen running water in his life, coming from the desert and all. Sure enough, right in the middle, with a small waterfall upstream and a big ugly hole downstream, Snake suddenly came uncoiled, and for a finale he fell into the hole upside down, with only his head and legs sticking out of the water.

"Dad yelled for Jep to cut loose the cans, and like lightning Jep bailed off his horse and was into the current with his knife. I'll tell you, there were a few tense moments while Jep tried to slice the lash ropes and Snake tried his damnedest to kick Jep's head off. Finally, however, Jep cut Snake loose, and the horse rolled over on his belly and eventually sloshed up our side of the bank, with Jep hanging off the side of the pack saddle like a wet gunny sack. The current had caught the fish cans and they started tumbling downstream, and soon both lids were off and hundreds of fingerling trout came boiling out. Some filtered into the lower pools, and others went streaking upstream to seek their fortunes there.

" 'Well,' said Jep once his teeth stopped chattering, 'you said we gotta change t' water!"

" 'Usually,' said Wonder real sarcastically, 'we do it with the fish in the can and not in the water.'

"Slim shrugged. 'Now how were we supposed to know that you wanted the fish left in the can? For a sophisticated operation like ours, you got to be more technical with your explanations.' And even the Wonder had to laugh.

"It was well after lunch by the time our pack train left the heavy timber along Swift Creek and started up through those high, open meadows towards Corner Peak. But we finally reached the base of the slide. I will admit that the slide and the wall above seemed to dwarf our pack train, and I had some serious second thoughts.

"We discussed it, and decided that given the loose surface of the slide, we'd have to lead the horses on foot, one at a time, and zigzag back and forth across the slope until we reached the gap. There, we'd have to unpack the horses and carry the fish cans on our backs through the crack. Then we could bring the horses up empty and repack 'em at the top. That was the plan, anyway, but you know what they say about the best-laid plans.

"Well, Jep started out with the first horse onto the scree, and I remember how each step caused a curtain of shale to slid down the embankment. Still, the first traverse went okay—that is, until the pack horse went to change directions on the switchback. The instant the horse turned uphill, the water sloshed downhill, and the weight of the fish cans pulled him backwards, and he lost his footing. It was a real bad scene! And there wasn't a damn thing any of us could do to stop it. We just stood there helplessly watching that poor animal doing somersaults, ass over teakettle, until he finally hit some boulders at the bottom of the slide and came to a stop. And of course, with each roll, the water from the cans spewed across the rock slide, leaving this glistening swath of fish flopping about on the hot rocks like stranded grunion!"

Casey shook his head. "It's a miracle that horse escaped without any broken bones, but he was sure bruised, and so scared that it took us two full hours just to coax him onto his feet and get him off the slide."

"My God!" Shag shook his head.

"Well, we weren't going to make the lake before night, that was clear. So Dad figured we'd better go back down a ways to the elk meadows, camp there and try the slide the next morning. Naturally, me being the youngest, I got stuck with the job of going back to the ranch for a tent and some supplies. But I didn't really mind. I was pretty discouraged since we'd lost a third of our fish stock and we still hadn't even crossed the slide. I just wanted to be alone. But all of a sudden, the Wonder remembered some reports back in town that required his attention—I think it was the sight of that horse falling ass over teakettle that jolted his memory. So he announced that he'd be going back with me.

" 'Maybe a soft bed and a warm woman sound good to Jep, too!' Jep teased.

"The Wonder tried to convince Jep that he'd be up half the night just writing the reports on those fish that got dumped into Swift Creek. 'And of course'—he nodded towards the scree field—'those.'

"But Jep ignored him, still thinking out loud that even a *warm* bed and a *soft* woman didn't sound bad. Before we left, Jep decided that since all he had waiting for him was a *hard* bed and a *cold* woman (or maybe a *cold* bed and a *hard* woman, he couldn't remember which), Jep would rather camp out in the mountains—provided he had some food.

" 'You make sure 'e comes back with some food,' Jep warned the Wonder. 'Otherwise, maybe we eat some fish from t'em cans. T'ey ain't so big so maybe we eat *lots*.'

"Anyway, I had a long ride ahead of me and I sure wasn't keen on baby-sitting the government man back to the ranch. 'You'd better keep up,' was all I said to him, and I started off at a lope down through the meadows and didn't slow down until we came to Swift Creek. Even then I didn't look back, and when I reached the other side, I set off again at a gallop. But you know, when I got to the ranch, I was in for the surprise of my life—the Wonder wasn't that far behind. Mind you, the guy was sure played right out, and when he finally rolled off his horse at the hitching rail, he just flopped down on the ground like a cloth doll and started talking to his legs like they weren't attached any more.

"I was in a hurry, and I kinda forgot about him and went on about my business. But pretty soon, would you believe, Millar came up to me and said he'd had a change of mind. He was going back with me! I told him I'd be all right, but he said those fish were his responsibility and he'd see them through to the lake. 'Suit yourself,' I told him.

"By the time I got all the supplies together, and fresh horses saddled, the sun was throwing long shadows off Terrace Peak. And of course, after Mom got through lecturing me about being careful going back in the dark, it *was* dark. Fortunately, the moon came up by the time we crossed Swift Creek and it was a beautiful night and I was actually a little sorry when we got to Dad's camp.

" 'The view ain't so bad—but the room service ain't worth an owl's hoot!' Dad said to me when I rode in. 'What kept you so long? Jep's already eaten the fish out of two cans,' he joked, 'and he's just starting on the third!' Then Slim saw the Wonder. 'Well, I'll be,' Dad said to him, 'you're a regular glutton for punishment, ain't you!' He shook his head mournfully, but you could tell he was impressed. 'Well, good, we're going to need every strong back and thick skull we can find.'

"Over breakfast the following morning, we discussed our predicament. It was obvious that a loaded pack horse couldn't pull the grade up the slide, let alone come through the gap. And since we were going to have to carry the milk cans on our backs through the break in the cliff anyway, we decided to hand pack them over the slide, too. Then we could bring the horses up empty, repack them on top and go on to the lake. Everyone figured we'd be home for supper.

"Well, as I recall, we ended up making our own packs out

of saddle pads, and with lash ropes tied through the handles, we had a harness that we could wear on our shoulders. That way each man could carry one can on his back and still have his hands free for balance. Even then you had to have help to getting started. And God save you if you stumbled, because you would either go bouncing like a loose bowling pin down the rockslide—which fortunately nobody did—or you'd fall uphill and be trapped like a turtle on its back until someone came along to roll you over.

"You can imagine, it was real slow going since every step you took in that loose shale, you'd slide back halfway. In fact, I remember Dad saying during one of our rests that climbing in that crap was the surest test of a man's commitment to fishing. At which point, Jep figured that since he only fished when he was hungry, and found no entertainment in catching them just for the sport of it, he'd gladly never eat another trout if we abandoned the project. Course, no one encouraged him and he grumbled that his mother didn't raise no dumb pack animals—but he kept on going like the rest of us dumb pack animals.

"For my part, I pretended I was Edmund Hillary—he was one of my heroes in those days. You know, suffering for a noble quest, driven by blind determination to conquer. At one point, I even fantasized that I was like Christ himself. Carrying my cross up a metaphorical Calvary, as if reaching the summit of the cliff would elevate me into angler martyrdom and guarantee me some rod room on the banks of a heavenly river." Casey chuckled. "But you know, when it finally got down to it, when eventually my imagination wore about as thin and raw as the skin on my back and hands, it was Millar who kept me going. I figured, hell, if he could do it, I could, too.

"And what's really funny, Millar told me later that he kept climbing because I did!" Casey paused, reflecting. "You know, in the last analysis, Millar turned out to be a pretty good man to have around, after all.

"Five hours to climb the rockslide, and another two hoisting the fish cans up through the split in the cliff. No sooner had we made the top and unpacked our loads than we noticed the neck of each can was plugged with a wad of dead fish. Which meant repacking the cans and hauling them another quarter-mile to change their water in a pool above the falls.

"But the *real* clincher was, we'd portaged only half our load; there were still four cans at the bottom of the slide, and the day was almost gone. Besides, we were way too tuckered out to make the climb again, especially by moonlight. But on the other hand, we couldn't just leave the cans there either... though Jep wasn't so sure.

"Finally, we decided to split the load. Dad and Millar would take the four cans at the bottom of the slide over to Ptarmigan Lake, which was a day's ride to the east. And at least you could get all the way in there on horseback. Jep and I would bring up the two strongest pack horses to the top, which turned out to be Whimples and Snake Bait, and then take the upper four cans of fish on to Cloud Lake.

"Course, by the time we scrambled down and returned with the two animals, it was too late to go any farther, so Jep and I picketed the horses in a small meadow back from the cliff and camped near the falls—if you can call it a camp." Casey snorted. "We were so tired out we didn't bother with supper or even pitching a tent. We just slept under our ponchos with the horse blankets to soften the rocks. Didn't even notice their smell—most likely we contributed to it.

"When I woke the next morning, the fog was so dense you couldn't see your hand at the end of your arm. And I wandered around for almost an hour looking for the picketed horses. Even then, I only found Whimples. Snake Bait must have learned to untie knots from the Shoshone, because he was long gone. Then Jep had some more good news.

" 'Tis morning we has a coyote breakfast!' he announced. 'We hurry so fast last night, you forget food.' "

"What's a coyote breakfast?" Sheila asked.

"Well, a coyote breakfast is a drink of water and a look around—and a deep breath if you're really hungry." Casey laughed. "In fact, the only good thing about a coyote breakfast is that it's easy to clean up afterwards. And let me tell you, Jep and I had a lot of them. Actually, however, that morning we were a little better off than usual. I had a small bag of coffee and an empty soup can in my saddlebag, and since neither of us was keen to ride around those cliffs blind in the fog, we stayed put and boiled coffee until the sun burned away the cover. Also, we had another problem that needed some figuring—there were four cans and only one pack horse. But after about the third helping of that embalming fluid we called coffee, Jep came up with the obvious solution—consolidate the fish into two cans. That way we could get by with only Whimples.

"Well, that's what we did, and just as soon as the sun came through, we saddled and packed Whimples and were on the trail. Still, after all the problems we'd had over the last two and a half days—especially since we'd figured the job would take only a day at most—I'd pretty well stopped believing we might really get the fish to the lake. Yet, as we reached that long meadow"—Casey nodded over his shoulder towards the meadow behind them—"I started thinking, by God, we're going to do it! Jep was feeling good, too, humming happy as a bumblebee in the warm sun and slapping his chaps to keep rhythm to his tune.

"Then, just as I could see the first thin profile of the lake edging out of the crater bottom, all hell broke loose!"

"Whimples?" asked Shag with anticipation.

"You guessed it. No more than a couple hundred yards short of the shoreline, Whimples decided she'd had enough! Which was just exactly why I didn't want her along in the first place . . . too goddamn unpredictable. And worst of all, when she'd throw a tizzy, she could buck the bandages off a mummy—hell, those fish cans were no challenge at all! The packsaddle rolled belly-under early into her routine. One can came completely loose and landed upside down in the outlet stream. The other one hung up in the lash ropes and bounced and banged along behind like a shivaree can tied to a newlywed's bumper—which, of course, just made Whimples even crazier.

"For me, it was the last straw. I started running after Whimples, throwing rocks the size of footballs. I'd've killed her if I could have hit her. Fortunately for her, I couldn't run very fast in my boots and chaps. Finally I got so damn mad and frustrated that I gave up chasing her and just pleaded with the Lord to kill her for me!

"Well, it was about then that I saw Jep out of the corner of my eye. He was down at the far end of the meadow, leaping about in the stream and flailing away at the water with a juniper limb like he'd been hit by ground hornets. I figured the Indian had finally lost his grip, until I saw what he was up to... Ol' Jep was driving those fingerlings up the stream towards the lake.

" 'T'ey 'erd real good!' Jep yelled, laughing like a little kid. 'Better t'en 'orses.'

"What the hell, I figured, and I started putting the minnows flopping around on the meadow moss into my hat and pitching them into the creek ahead of Jep. When we got the first batch to the lake, we ran back downstream and started up with another wave of stragglers. Back and forth, for nearly two hours, trying to salvage what we could from Whimples's wreckage, And eventually"—Casey sighed—"even Whimples, damn her hide.

" 'Course, nobody'll believe it,' Jep said when it was all over, " 'cept you and me, cuz everyone knows you's a liar... and me's an Indian!'

"And since we figured the venture was a write-off, no one bothered to tell the government the final details. In fact, we kinda forgot about the fish, until maybe five years later when I was hunting near here and curiosity got the best of me." Casey stopped and looked at his audience.

"Now, I ain't saying that those fish"—he nodded towards Shag's catch—"are related to the ones Jep and I herded. And I will say, the fry Dad and Millar planted in Ptarmigan Lake survived real well. So who knows." He smiled at Sheila and Shag. "Maybe some of them *did* come over the mountain."

Then Casey leaned forwards and scooped the charred scraps of fish skin out of the frying pan into the fire. A nighthawk peeled across the mountain basin, destined for a nocturnal hunting foray in the valley below. If Casey listened carefully to the sounds beyond the outlet stream sweeping across the gravel shoals, he could hear, far in the distance, the tenor thunder of the waterfall cascading over the great cliff.

"Well! There you are." He smiled. "You can weigh the evidence and decide for yourself which theory is true."

For a long time they sat in silence, looking across the lemon-coloured lake as the stars pranced with impunity upon its surface. In the crystal air, the two black, gnarly, giant peaks seemed to surge and then retreat back and forth against the horizon.

"Tomorrow," Shag said, "show me that ridge the trout migrated over."

SHOEING ON THE SABBATH

BUDDY LOOKED LIKE A FEEDING FLAMINGO AS HE BENT OVER THE horse's elevated hoof, using his legs for a table so his hands were free to do the shoeing. Sweat soaked his sleeveless shirt down to where it disappeared under the belt of his chaps. Sweat ran off his brow into his eyes, making them sting and blurring his vision. It tracked down the bridge of his nose, welling into droplets that splashed onto the bottom of the horse's desert-dry hoof. Buddy didn't know what he wanted to be—just fifteen years old, he had lots of time to decide—but he was sure he could scratch farrier from his list. He would shoe for the family, Buddy decided, for kin and blood, but never for wages!

Under any other circumstance it would have been a beautiful day. A water day, for lying in the lake or floating on an inner tube down the river trolling for trout. But if you had to shoe horses, it definitely was not a good day. Not even noon and already the air was heavy and motionless like a crushing blanket suffocating the valley bottom and the horse corrals. Even the dust, when it chose to rise at all, puffed listlessly and collapsed like a tired old hunting dog. Still, it was the only time Slim could spend with Buddy teaching him to shoe, what with the guests and running the ranch and all.

Slim squatted near his grandson. Consolidated under the shade of his cowboy hat, he looked like a bird balanced on a rock. His arms were folded around his knees, though his hands hung out in the sun, ready to pass Buddy a tool or illustrate a story with a map of some distant valley drawn in the dust. He'd measured his perch from his grandson, close enough for consultation but still out of the way of an errant hoof, or a flying shoer on the end of an errant hoof. Not that there was much chance of old Lightning striking out.

Lightning, named for a jagged swipe of white hair across the horse's otherwise black hide (and certainly not for any reserves of bolt energy), dozed on three legs and depended heavily upon Buddy's back for the fourth point of contact. Horseflies and deerflies, ferocious with the sun and the abundance of succulent horse and human flesh, swarmed like threatening fighter planes, circling for a tactical strike between sweeps of the horse's tail, on a narrow target of exposed skin above Buddy's collar.

Whap! Lightning's tail swung at a fly, catching Buddy in the face.

"Damn you, nag! If you're not careful" Buddy growled at the sleeping horse, "I'll stake you out for bear bait!"

Slim began to laugh, and the wrinkles of weathered flesh around his eyes creased like deep folds in a well-worn comforter. "Once this fella and me was shoeing down in old Mexico—south of Santa Rosa, as best I recall. But I do remember it was a hot day like today and the flies was buzzing thick like now, and just like Lightning done to you there, this partner of mine gets his face slapped a few times. Well, this guy figures he'll put a stop to that real quick, and he ties a shoeing hammer to the end of the horse's tail so it can't swing!"

Buddy looked skeptically at Slim.

"Gospel! Saw it for myself." Slim grinned, turning up his open hands, maybe to prove he had nothing up his sleeve. "Well, don't you know, the very next horsefly that comes along left my partner unconscious for the better part of the afternoon!"

Buddy started laughing, breaking the delicate equilibrium between shoer and shod. He tried to stagger free of Lightning and drop the horse's foot to the ground, but without its crutch, the animal jolted awake off balance and fell towards Buddy, stepping on the side of the boy's boot. "Damn you, Lightning!" Buddy slapped the horse's rump with his bare hand, serving only to make his hand sting with no noticeable effect upon the horse.

Gingerly Buddy straightened. With his hands on his hips, he arched backwards, stretching the muscles that had been painfully knotted from the horse's weight. He unbuckled his shoeing chaps and laid them across the anvil before moving awkwardly into the shade of the saddle shed. A gallon mayonnaise jar of cold water lay in the thick timothy grass. Beads of condensation shimmered on the glass like opals. Beside it the curly-haired black dog, Jude, chewed rapturously on scraps of horse's hoof. Buddy spun the lid on the jar and offered Slim first drink.

"Go ahead." Slim waved off the container. "I'm just the helper on this job. You're the working man now."

Buddy felt a pulse of pride. Taking the jar in both hands, he drank from the rim, letting the water slop around the edges of his mouth and run off his chin onto his chest. Finally he sat down heavily in the shade beside Slim. He had to admit, it felt good being included in the work, the real work. Previous years he'd been just the "catch and fetch," holding the horses, handing the cowboys tools as they needed them.

"You're still slow as a glacier," Slim teased, "but you're getting the hang of it. One more hoof and we'll have to stop and go fishing." He drew out his gold pocket watch and opened the cover. "Eleven-thirty. Your grandma will be back from church soon and she'd have a tizzy-fit if she caught us shoeing on the Sabbath."

"Grandpa," Buddy asked after some time thinking, "what's your religion?"

The question startled Slim. He looked at Buddy, trying to see what was behind it. "You figure I'd be naked without one?" Slim asked. Then he grinned. "I guess, if I got one, it's trout fishing. A clear trout stream is about as inspirational as any church I've ever seen.

"Besides, son, don't you know that too much religion ain't healthy? Take your great-uncle Whitney, for instance. Boy-howdy! I never know'd a person so festered up about sin and suffering. And, by gosh, in the end, he up and died from it!" Slim let the sentence dangle before pulling the line. "That's right. Went to church *twice* in one day, if you can imagine, and on the second dose he got run over by a Model T delivery truck. He'd probably still be alive," Slim added with exaggerated sobriety, "if he'd been satisfied with the normal measure, instead of trying to double-time it to the Pearlies." Slim snorted. "But I guess he got there twice as fast, and I suppose the Lord was impressed."

"Sounds to me like the delivery truck was to blame for working on the Sabbath." Buddy smiled. "But I thought you were Mormon?"

"Well, between you, me and the gatepost"—he glanced around as if someone might be listening—"I don't hold much store in *any* religion!"

This surprised Buddy. He'd always assumed Slim, like Ethel (or likely because of Ethel), was Mormon. His grandparents seemed to think with one mind. Or maybe they just didn't discuss their differences.

"What you got against religion?" Buddy prodded.

Again Slim stared at the boy thoughtfully. "For one thing, most religions spend a good chunk of their time peddling their wares. It seems to me like the truth should sell itself and it don't need vendors. Anyway, some things—like faith, for instance—don't mean squat unless you find them yourself. Besides, you can't teach faith, you got to feel it inside you."

Slim sat there quietly. "And for another thing," he added after some thought, "most religions put too much stock in God meddling in man's affairs—'working miracles' as your grandma says. In fact, sometimes I think they figure God exists just for *their* fetching! No, sir, to my way of thinking, wishing for miracles is like asking God to do our chores cause we're too lazy to do them ourselves. Besides, hoping for miracles drains off energy you could spend helping yourself or even helping others." Slim reflected for a moment. "Who knows, maybe God expects *us* to do the miracles!"

Buddy wasn't sure about that. For him, the most interesting stories in Sunday school were the miracles. They were magic, a great magician feeding the multitude, retrieving Lazarus from the dead. Surely Lazarus couldn't do that himself.

"You don't believe that Jesus worked miracles?" he asked.

Slim rubbed his chin. "About as much as I believe anything somebody tells me who wasn't there. Oh, don't get me wrong," he added, "I ain't saying Jesus weren't inspired by God. But then, a lot of folks is inspired, ain't they? Some even say Johnny Nisbett's inspired."

"Johnny Nisbett!" Buddy squawked. "He isn't inspired—he's crazy!"

"Well, he claims he's got God's ear and that the communication line's working in both directions."

"So you're saying Jesus was crazy?" Buddy felt uncomfortable with the terrain. He'd never heard anyone speak against Christ, except maybe to use his name when swearing, but that was small measure compared to calling him insane!

"Let me ask you this, son, do the things Jesus taught seem crazy?" Slim asked. Buddy thought for a moment and shook his head.

"Then if what he said's the truth, what difference does it make if he had all his wits about him or if he'd just been shoeing donkeys for too long in the open sunshine?"

Buddy guessed that Slim was baiting him to do his own thinking. He decided to let the hook rest. "I'd better finish Lightning before Grandma comes back." He scruffed the black dog and bolted upright. Lobster hot, he thought, boiling, lobster-pot hot. He locked onto the rhythm of the phrase as he lifted Lightning's last leg. "Lobster-pot hot, you overdue bear bait, lobster-pot hot!"

"So what's got you to thinking about God and all?" Slim followed him out into the furnace.

"Well, you always said my brain outran my feet."

"But not always your mouth," Slim teased him and handed Buddy the hoof knife. Buddy began cleaning the dirt and gravel from the thick sides of the frog, cutting off the scales of leather-tough skin.

"This morning at breakfast, Grandma set me to wondering," Buddy said. "The way she fretted about me not going to church with her. You know she wants to marry you in the Salt Lake Temple so you'll be man and wife in heaven?"

Slim looked bewildered; he hadn't heard. "Can't!" He

finally shook his head. "Already spoken for. She should'a asked sooner!" He warmed to the unfolding joke. "'Sides, I can't marry just any Sadie come lately, not for eternity, leastways."

"Sadie come lately!" Buddy smirked. "You've been married to her for forty years!"

"Well, the truth is"—Slim's brow furrowed—"I doubt that any ceremony heaped in all that gold and red carpet and all is any better than a simple sage-chicken wedding in front of a prairie preacher." The man shifted on his haunches, again crossing his arms over his knees. "Just remember, on the back of a rank bronc, a silver-plated saddle ain't gonna ride no better than a rough leather one. Anyway, Buddy, marriage ain't about where or how you was tied, it's how you respect each other afterwards that sticks two people together. Oh, I'll probably do it, just to stop her infernal badgering," he said with a sigh of resignation, "but she'll have to ask proper!"

Buddy realized they'd wandered far off the subject of Slim's religion without getting to the meat of the matter. "Grandpa, if you don't have a religion, do you believe in God?"

"What?" Slim sounded like a startled gander. "You still holding onto that line?" He stared at Buddy. Then the edges of his mouth turned up. "Your grandma says I must cuz I use God's name so much."

"No, seriously, Grandpa?" Buddy asked.

"Sure." Slim shrugged. "Just because a person don't have a pedigree religion don't mean he can't believe in something, does it?" Slim traced the outline of his boots in the dust with his finger. "Son, I'll tell you the truth about religion and me. It seems like religion is just a sack for holding all the church's hoopla. But if your faith don't need the headdresses and the buffalo robes and all, then you probably don't need a religion to pack them around in."

Slim pointed at the side of Lightning's hoof. "Look here, son, now don't cut so deep with the nips. You won't be able to set the nails without quicking him."

Buddy adjusted the bite of the hoof nippers to where Slim pointed and began clipping the cuticle. A twist of hoof peeled away like an orange rind. The moment the helix hit the ground, Jude darted in, grabbed it and trotted off with his head high and proud like a cannibal with a fat thigh bone.

Buddy waited for his grandpa to return to the topic, but the man was absorbed with Jude's antics.

"Why?" Buddy asked finally.

"Why what?"

"Why do you believe in God?"

Slim studied the boy dubiously. "Why do I believe in God?" Slim decided to be straight with Buddy. "Too many things we can't explain," he said sincerely, "and too much organization behind them, once we do figure them out."

"What things?"

"Well . . ." Slim raised his hand, flexing the fingers, drawing his thumb and index together. "That, for one."

Again Buddy was unsure of Slim's point. "You mean, the way the body works?" The boy raised his head with the question. "Nowadays, biology has solved almost all the mystery around that." Buddy's biology teacher had said it first.

Slim hummed pensively, considering Buddy's comment. "Solved?" He smirked. "Seems to me that every answer I've ever found always led me to another question. But I guess your science is different." Slim picked up a stone, spit on it, then polished it on his pants leg. "I think if a person really looks at something close, he can't help but find the hand of God someplace along the line. Take, for sake's sake, our brains. Now from what I gather, which ain't much, ideas don't just bang around in there like a bunch of billiard balls. There's order to them, they lead from one to the next. All I'm saying is, no matter how far scientists go, they always discover that Mother Nature's organized." He rolled the stone between his thumb and forefinger. "And I guess to my way of thinking, you could say a science book is just as much about God as, say, the Bible or Ethel's *Book of Mormon*!"

Slim studied the rock. It was blood-red with thin wafers of white quartz running through in perfectly parallel waves. "But I doubt seriously that they'll ever whittle *everything* down to just nuts and bolts in a machine . . . not everything. For instance, how does your scientist explain something that you can't put your hands on, like feelings or imagination? Where do they come from? Or take something really slippery. What about something like beauty?" Slim held up the rock for Buddy to see. "Like a sunrise, or say this here rock?"

Buddy glanced up.

"Because you see, it ain't so much that nature's beautiful." Slim rolled the stone in his fingers, following the waves. "The real miracle is that we got in our head what it takes to see it, and feel it, and get inspired by it. Now that's the real miracle!"

"I thought you didn't believe in miracles," Buddy teased.

Slim smiled and studied the rock. Then a thought occurred to him. "Even if we could answer every how that there is to creation, Buddy, we still ain't any closer to the root of the matter." Slim paused. "Did you ever think, *why* creation? That's the real winning question, ain't it? *Why* is there life at all, when so much is working agin it?"

Suddenly an idea amused Slim. "I've heard some folks say that creation came about by chance, like me taking apart my watch and shaking the pieces in that feedbag yonder till eventually they all came together and it'd start ticking! To my way of thinking, that don't make no sense at all—and that's just a watch! What's more, somebody had to do the shaking, and there's still the question of why."

He looked at Buddy. "Nope," he said with a note of finality, "there's too many things we can't explain—and too much sense behind them when we do find an explanation." He opened the palms of his hands. "So, that's why I figure there's a God!"

Buddy drove the burred face of a rasp across the bottom of the hoof, showering the ground with a snowstorm of white scrapings. He understood how a person could have faith without religion, though somehow it *did* make a difference to him if Christ were sane or crazy. The truth was, however, Buddy knew well what Slim was talking about, and he suspected that the seed of his own interest in biology was planted by Slim's acute sense of awe for nature.

"So, what's your God like?" Buddy asked.

Slim frowned and shook his head with exaggerated pain. "Son, you're a regular glutton for punishment, ain't you! Sure you really want to go after this? Your grandmammy gets wind that I've been preaching heathen ideas to you"—he drew a finger like a knife across his throat—"and she'll have both our hides tanning on the tabernacle wall before sunset."

"I won't repeat a word, may old Lightning here strike me down!"

"And I wouldn't go taunting either ol' Lightning or the Lord if I was you."

"What *do* you think He's like?" Buddy persisted.

"You sure God's a He?" Slim removed his Stetson and scrubbed his sleeve across his brow. "Ain't it possible God's a She? Or maybe like the Shoshone believe, God's a They. You know Indians believe in a whole passel of gods!"

Buddy had never considered God as anything except He. Masculine, unshaven, old yet ageless, wise enough to somehow move rocks bigger than Himself and be two places at once, patient like Slim but not so much fun. Buddy was suddenly surprised. If he looked hard at his idea of God, He was humourless, passionless and bland as pancake batter, as Slim would say.

"What would you suppose," Slim went on, "if God is just an *it*! In fact, what if God was *every* it that you can imagine—everything! And what if everything that is, and was, and will be is just part of God?" He paused, letting the question ride. "Maybe what we call things are just globs of the same goop? The sagebrush, that timbered ridge yonder, that horsefly on the back of your neck." Seemingly alerted that his presence had been discovered, the fly bit fast and hard before Buddy could react. Slim sucked on his lower lip to keep from laughing.

"God damn it!" Buddy rubbed the bite for a moment. "I can't for the life of me fathom the god-goop bullshit in horseflies!"

"Well, if God is everything, then even flies got some measure of it in them."

The horsefly gave focus to Buddy's frustration. He was hot and tired, and once again he didn't understand what Slim was getting at. "The Bible says God created everything. You mean like everything comes from God?" he asked hopefully.

"Hmm. Not comes from, more like everything that's been

created *is* God." Slim's eyes twinkled. "God ain't someplace *else* where you got to call long distance."

"Grandpa?" Buddy really wasn't sure if he should ask. "Do you pray?"

"Not enough to say so," he said, flipping the rock he'd been playing with into the air. It sailed high, landing in the corral dust with a soft *plump*.

Buddy was again astonished. He'd never thought of Slim as *not* praying! Though when he tried to picture the man down on his knees, he got instead Slim squatting on his haunches, talking straight to God as though the two of them had just come off the river and were discussing what they'd caught and how they'd done it. Buddy laughed. Slim swapping lies with the Lord.

Slim handed him the last horseshoe off the corral rail. But after all the time Buddy had taken rasping the bottom of the foot, the shoe still rocked at the heels. If it wasn't set right, it would drop off in couple weeks.

"Here, son, just file a little more off the toe. That's all it takes." Slim showed him where to rasp, and this time the shoe rested flat and steady. He handed Buddy a few shoeing nails. "Remember, always turn the scored face of the nail in, so the point'll come out of the hoof." Slim showed him how to bend the tip of the nail and set it with a slight outward slope. "One bad nail can sure cripple a horse."

Buddy stuck a nail into the shoe and began hammering, but no sooner had he set one and started to drive a second than Slim stopped him in mid-swing.

"Whoa, there!" he barked. "Never start the second nail till you've twisted the point off the first. If your horse jumps, that nail will shred your leg like a bear claw done it."

Again he fell silent. "I prayed once," he confessed after watching the boy work for a while "the time your daddy shot his arm off and your uncle Reg come down to the ranch to fetch me. Going back in to town on the sleigh that night I prayed. Boy-howdy, did I pray!" His eyes glazed as he focussed on the memory. "But you know, son, in the last tally, I seen that it was Casey who'd have to fight the fight. He'd have to heal himself and bring himself along with just one arm."

Suddenly Slim's eyes sparkled again. "Naw, I figure praying is too close to begging. 'Sides, there's a lot folks got problems bigger than any of mine. They can take my place in line."

"But aren't you concerned about heaven?" Buddy asked.

"Heaven?" Slim thought for a moment. "Ever notice, Buddy, how some folks make themselves just miserable, figuring they'll be happy later in heaven? It seems to me a lot smarter to get the most we can out of *this* life and be pleasantly surprised if there's something after than to go moping around like a gutshot elk, only to find that the Pearlies is closed for repairs anyway. Nope," Slim said firmly, "I don't give much to them that goes on all sorry-faced, believing that God's going to thump their butts for enjoying being alive." Again he was rolling with the humour of the idea. "Like some churches, they'd sooner crucify you than let you dance. Can you imagine?"

Buddy loved to watch Slim and Ethel dance. "I got two left feet," Slim would say, "and Ethel's got two right! We're a perfect match!" They were graceful, even regal, when the accordion and fiddle band played a slow porcelain waltz. But let the band hit upon a polka, and Buddy's grandparents were like orbiting, spinning planets, their heels swinging high in the air like comets in hot pursuit of the couple twirling in great circles around the dance-hall galaxy.

"Seems to me, dancing is a whole lot closer to godliness than crying and whipping yourself, like some Christians still do, over something that happened two thousand years ago to a bunch of folks you ain't even related to!"

Slim fell silent for a moment, considering his words. "Buddy, did you ever think . . . what if the only way God gets to dance is through us?"

Buddy glanced up to see if Slim was kidding him again. To the boy's surprise, his grandfather was rock earnest.

"Just suppose, for the sake of supposing, that maybe that's our job here on earth . . . to live for God."

Finally Buddy thought he understood. "Doing God's bidding, like Grandma says?" "Hardly! That's just living by somebody else's rules. No, what I mean is something different." He thought for a moment. "Maybe God sees Itself through our eyes. Maybe, son, that's our purpose—to be God's mirror!"

Slim saw he'd lost Buddy completely. "Seems like I've overloaded your plate, son. It ain't really important that you understand now. Chew on the ideas for a while." Slim rose. "Listen, Buddy, I don't really know nothing for sure. 'Sides, a person can't teach *or* preach God. You just got to feel it."

Slim showed Buddy how to pull Lightning's foot forward and turn it so the boy could rest it face down on his knee, then file the upper edge of the hoof to the contour of the shoe. When Buddy had finished, Slim gave the hoof a final inspection and tapped Buddy on the shoulder. "Let her rip!"

This time Buddy pushed back against the horse instead of dropping the hoof.

"Wake up, thunderbolt!" he barked. Again the horse jolted awake, but this time on four legs. One leg, however, was still asleep, and again Lightning fell against Buddy, stepping on the side of his boot. Stumbling away from the weight of the horse, Buddy straightened his muscles and again the needles of pain shot up his back. Never, never for wages, he resolved.

Buddy looked long at the sun, then at his grandfather. "So that's it?" he asked. "Dance for God?"

"Plus maybe fish for trout, and don't tie a shoeing hammer to a horse's tail during fly season!" Slim laughed. "What more does a person need to know?"

Slim spied a distant funnel of dust coming up the road on the other side of the river. "Your grandma's on her way home; best put the horse away and pick up your tools. And mind yourself," he added, "don't tell her what's been going on here or she'll have your butt in church till the pew wears a hole in your hide."

"When's she going to nail our hides to the tabernacle wall?"

"That'll come next, after your soul's been chewed soft like moccasin leather!" He caught Buddy with his eyes to punctuate the sinister warning. "Come on, Jude," Slim called to the dog, "we'll go intercept her." He glanced around at the dog. "Jude! Put that down! She'll catch us for sure!" Obediently the dog dropped the piece of horse's hoof and padded up the hill after the man.

SATURDAY NIGHT

"WELL I'M A HONKY-TONK MAN!" EARL'S OFF-KEY TENOR challenged Johnny Horton on the radio. "And I can't seem to stop. I love to give the girls a whirl to the music of an old jukebox." Earl beat out the rhythm on the pickup's steering wheel, weaving the old Chevrolet down the winding canyon road towards town. "And when my money's all gone, I'm on the telephone, saying, 'Hey, hey, Mama, can your daddy come home?'"

Buddy watched as Earl drew his hat down just above his eyes and let out a low wolf howl. It had been a long week for the cowboys. The range grass was drying out early this year, and the main herd of cows kept pressing into alpine valleys, which were thick with deadly lupine and larkspur. Every hour of every day, someone had been in the saddle holding the cattle back. Ah, Buddy thought, but that was then, and now is bathed and shaved, a white shirt and a good hat. Saturday night and they'd just got paid.

Riding herd on cows, Buddy decided, was still a lot better than riding herd on dudes. "Peopled out," Slim had called it. He was the one who suggested that Buddy take a break from the guest ranch and try a season of range riding. Buddy heard that the foreman at the Double J was looking for help, and Earl had hired him on the spot.

"Oh, my soul's woeful full of silence." Earl growled like a cougar. "I need me a hank of hair and a hunk of tail."

Earl was different from the quiet cowboys Buddy had been raised with. He was rough and unruly—qualities Buddy wanted to cultivate. For a cowboy in his early fifties, Earl was still Hollywood handsome: an angular face with a strong, jutting chin and heavy, brooding, sash-curtain eyelids. Buddy knew all too well that his friend's good looks were both a curse and a blessing. The blessing was that women were always after Earl's attention. Unfortunately, they all too often came with jealous boyfriends, who were equally anxious to rearrange Earl's face to a more equitable standard. Buddy saw it was a bad combination because Earl couldn't turn down either a lady or a fight. And a couple of times Buddy had been caught in the middle.

Sandwiched between Buddy and Earl sat Taylor. He was a large, beefy man in his mid-twenties, with an obtrusive brow that betrayed laboured thinking. He was a Kansas farm boy who got strung out on the rodeo merry-go-round, and like all cheap-thrill addicts, Buddy suspected, he didn't know how or when to get off. "The lights are on," Earl would tease Taylor, "but nobody's home!"

That night, like every Saturday night throughout the summer, Taylor's thick concentration was locked on the saddle bronc he'd drawn at the rodeo: spur high, stay loose, reach and lean forward like sitting in a rocking chair. He rocked forward and back in the truck, draining the last of the Coors from a can in the process. He crushed the container and pitched it onto the floor, adding to the truck's permanent carpet of flattened beer cans.

"Say, you better take it easy, Flash," Earl cautioned Taylor. "You got a horse to ride and a long night of tonk'n after that."

Taylor gave Earl a cold look and defiantly snapped another tab.

"And for those of you new to the area," the honey voice of the radio disk jockey intoned , "let me remind you of our Wild West show on the town square, seven o'clock tonight and every night. It's an authentic slice from our colourful past. Don't miss it, pardner. See you there!"

"What a crock of shit!" Earl snorted. "If those marshmallow show boys had tamed the Old West, we'd still be sitting with the Indians in wigwams, smoking peace pipes and eating buffalo meat. About the only one in the whole show that's believable is Tulip!"

Buddy never did have much use for Tulip Meeker. In the first place Tulip wasn't his name, it was Two-lip, a nickname he'd acquired because his lips peeled back in a perpetual sneer. And secondly there was the missing firewood incident. In fact, in Buddy's opinion, Tulip was just a bar stool cowboy whose bent for larceny and lechery was fortunately kept in check by an equal lack of ambition, rendering him, in the final equation, a harmless nuisance.

The one job Tulip seemed perfect for was Black Bart in the Wild West show. For, besides his perpetual sneer and his dark personality in general, the single quality that assured him a role in the nightly street theatre was the ominous black patch hiding an ugly eye socket—punctured, it was said, by a wild piece of kindling in a chopping shed. His job was to rob the stage and drool over the pretty passengers long enough for the sheriff to catch him. The posse would threaten to hang him, but always in the end there would be a shoot out, and Tulip would end up slabbed over his horse like a side of beef and hauled off into the sunset—only to be resurrected like Lazarus for the following night's performance.

"Should'a hung him years ago!" Earl groused.

"I think he stole some firewood off us one time," said Buddy. "Least someone took it, and every time I'd see him afterwards, he'd look guilty as stink with that one eye spooking around at everything 'cept me."

"Hell, that don't mean he's guilty. That's the way that eye is all the time. Like maybe it's got more control than the man behind it."

"More likely, he's light-fingered something from everybody in town and can't look *nobody* in the eye. That's my guess."

"Humph," Earl snorted. "The ol' blue-haired gals sure think he's honey on their toast. Two of them was buying him drinks last Saturday in the Cowboy. Say, that reminds me of a joke." Everything reminded Earl of a joke. "Did you hear the one about the two old maids that went on a drunk? No? Well, they almost killed him!"

Buddy laughed, but Taylor frowned. "I don't get it. I thought you said they went on a drunk. Who's him?"

"A drunk!" Earl turned his hand in front of Taylor's face,

trying to show him the twist of the word. "A drunk...a drunk!"

"Screw you," Taylor sneered, "I still don't get it."

Earl didn't bother any more and looked over at Buddy. "The fact remains, somebody'd do the world a big favour if they'd put Tulip out of his suffering." Then an idea struck Earl as funny. "Somebody should stick real bullets in those show boys' guns!"

"Wouldn't that be a hoot?" Buddy chuckled.

"Sheriff Bow never would figure out what happened. Probably arrest one of the actors."

"Or one of the tourists!" Taylor's laugh came in puffs like wind off a fan blade.

Bow had been sheriff of Skyline for as long as Buddy could remember, probably because no one else ever ran for the job. There wasn't any crime to mention in Skyline, and Bow's main occupations seemed to be keeping track of his three renegade daughters and halting the downward pull of his gun belt as it tried to drag his pants from his hips.

Finally, across the valley, the lights of town began to dance before them like a Vegas show girl shimmering seductively in the thick summer twilight. By day, the town was hardly noticeable snuggled beneath a row of talon-shaped mountains that hooked abruptly out of the valley floor. Once it was exclusively a cow town, but the mountains brought tourists, and even in Buddy's short memory, Skyline had changed considerably. The harness shop became a land developer's office, and Watson's Mercantile became Watson's Western Art Gallery. In the end, it seemed to Buddy, about the only things unchanged were the bars and their dwindling legion of patrons. Still, for a lonely, horny cowboy, Skyline's blemishes were easily missed in the radiance of promise. Earl had got them dates with women from the Suds-R-Us laundry, friends of Elsie, Earl's "regular." Buddy leaned forward with anticipation. "Well, I'm a honky-tonk man," he sang and pulled his hat down low like Earl's.

"Hey, pretty mama!" Earl grabbed Elsie just outside the Tumbleweed Bar, giving her a wagon-wheel swing that scattered the startled tourists off the wooden boardwalk. Regaining herself, she playfully cuffed his ears, then, performing for the wide-eyed passers-by, she threw her arms around his neck and gave him a wild, audible kiss.

Buddy looked at the two women with Elsie. The short one was plump, with hair blacker than her complexion suggested was natural. She had a pretty face, round and wholesome in spite of the heavy-handed attempts at worldliness with eyeliner and lipstick. Buddy thought she might be what Earl called flypaper, a woman looking for a man to reform.

The other women didn't wear make up. She was not that tall, though her long brunette hair, which hung below her shoulders, made her seem so. While her face was open and rather plain, she had long cattail eyelashes sheltering blue, watery eyes. But it was the dress that held Buddy's attention. It was Christmas-wrapping red, a tight-knit weave that contoured to her body, following each movement like a lonely cat. Buddy guessed that she was older than him by a few years. Normally that would have been enough to rein back his shaky confidence around her . . . if it weren't for the dress. He gave her a big, stupid smile as if he was posing for a portrait.

"Where are my manners?" Elsie apologized. "This is Melody and Betty Sue." Melody, the lady in red, smiled warmly at Buddy. She, too, had made her choice.

"Melody? I never met a real Melody," Buddy said, keeping the moronic grin for safety.

"Well," she erupted with an embarrassed giggle, "you still haven't! It's actually Mary, but I changed it for the summer."

"Melody suits you just fine! I'm Alexander, but they call me Buddy."

The entrance of the Tumbleweed Bar was choked with tourists and want-to-be cowboys. Earl, in the lead, pressed his way in and wove through the crowded dance floor to find room in the rear, with the "authentic colour," as Earl called his friends.

"Whooee!" he yelled above the bar noise. "The R Lazy S gang! Better known to their mothers as 'our lazy asses.'" At a round table sat a half dozen cowboys and girls. Earl grabbed one of the men by the shoulder. Jackson was a big man, slightly Earl's junior. He wore a bright floral western shirt pulled taut across his barrel chest. He had a jocular face and a

Fuller brush moustache pruned like a longhorn at the ends. The crease of his hat was down the centre in a style from a century past.

"How are your lazy asses?" Earl gave him a pat on the back.

"Damnation!" wailed Jackson, "if it ain't Elder Earl himself!" Elder was a nickname for Earl, earned by his fondness for preaching whenever he had hard drink and a captive audience. "Pull up some chairs and put a load on your minds." Jackson gestured around the table. "Know everyone?"

Next to Jackson was an olive-skinned woman wearing a beaded chamois-skin shirt. Instead of sleeves, long strands of fringe dangled down her sun-browned arms. Her face was framed by braids. Buddy first thought she was a mixed breed, until he discovered that she came from the East. A Radcliffe girl who was more western than most women raised in the Rockies. Which was good, since she was the cook at the R Lazy S, plus Jackson's lady, both tasks demanding a strong frontier spirit.

Across the table from them sat two cowhands. One was so drunk that he still hadn't zeroed in on them, and his eyes ranged back and forth like a camera lens trying to focus. The other one was too obsessed playing back-up percussion on the table top to the band's electric "bomp-sha-bomp" to realize the gang had grown.

At the far end of the table was an Indian, an Arapaho from the east slope. Buddy knew him only as Fireweed. Supposedly he was once a shaman in a hippie commune, hence his name. He was a heavy-set man with shoulder-length black hair and an unnatural smile. Only the eyes moved in the Buddha face, watching and weighing the scene. Everything's fine, the eyes said. And if everything was fine with you, that was fine with Fireweed. However, should conditions change and become just ever so slightly not to Fireweed's liking, he generally went snaky crazy. Which was fine, too . . . as long as Buddy was out of the way!

"So, everybody, this is Melody and Betty Sue, and you know Elsie." Earl introduced the women. The R Lazy S crew nodded like feeding chickens.

"What happened to you last Saturday night? I thought you were coming in" Earl said. "We hit every brew joint in Skyline looking for you, including the tourist traps."

"Well, Elder Earl, seems we had our own party," Jackson replied, "moving cows out of the high country up the Crystal Creek divide and then pushing them all the way down to the Gros Vente meadows. Damnation, was it cold for August!" Jackson turned to his girl friend. "Sure wish I had my Radcliffe squaw. As it was, I had to sleep all night with my wangle in my hand just to keep it from freezing solid!"

"I told you I should have come," the woman with braids teased.

"So, Buddy, you finally found yourself a woman," Jackson said looking at Melody. Buddy cringed. "And now you figure you're gonna finally get laid?" Jackson asked, causing Buddy to turn red with embarrassment and anger.

"Say, Taylor, you rodeoing tonight?" Jackson turned his attention to the other cowboy with Earl

"You're a rodeo rider?" asked Betty Sue, her eyes wide with admiration. "I've never seen a rodeo. Could I come along? Maybe I'll bring you luck!"

Taylor's grin was as wide as a barn door, and an open one, at that, for he was missing four front teeth. Only once before had a woman been there to watch him ride. It was in El Paso, when he won first-prize money in the bareback event. He didn't see her after the rodeo, since they took him immediately to Emergency to have his right shoulder pinned together. Unfortunately, Taylor's lady was holding his truck keys. The Royal Canadian Mounted Police found his pickup in Alberta two weeks later.

Earl reached into his jeans pocket and handed Taylor the keys to the Chevrolet. "You hang onto them this time, and if there's any winnings, bring 'em back and we'll let you pay for the night's drinking!"

"Fifteen minutes before showtime, folks—a slice out of the Old West !" squawked a loud-speaker truck on the street.

Earl wagged his head in disgust. "Calling the lambs to slaughter."

"Calling the heathen to hell is closer to the truth," Jackson grumbled. "You ask me, this place was a whole lot better when it was a cow town instead of a damn tourist trap. And the height of their stupidity,"—he shook a finger towards the door—"is that damn street circus. If I could figure out a way, I'd shut down that nonsense real fast."

"Hell, if a plan's all you're lacking...." Earl grinned.

Buddy shifted in his chair uneasily. When Jackson and Earl got together, even the best plans often turned, as Earl called it, "wild, woolly and a wee bit western." It was as if neither of them had a solid grasp on the limits of propriety, or even safety, for that matter.

"Do you dance?" Buddy asked Melody, anxious to avoid being coralled into Jackson's and Earl's scheme.

She smiled. "Whenever I get the chance."

The drummer started a heavy cadence into "Pretty Woman." Melody caught the beat and snapped her ass in the red dress as she strutted through the tables like a young colt stretching its legs on spring pasture.

"Mercy!" moaned the vocalist.

"Mercy!" Buddy echoed in a soft, guttural growl, watching the woman throw back her mane and beckon to him. Buddy followed, wondering if this was to be *the night*.

A crowd of tourists had gathered at Skyline's main intersection, where it formed the corner of the town square. The square was actually a park facing four streets of western storefronts, disguising the curio shops, resturants and bars, like the Tumbleweed. Originally, it was where you tied your horses and parked your wagon when you came to town for supplies. Now it was a quiet oasis from the summer's exhausting pursuit of capitalism. One corner of the park, the one facing the main intersection, had an archway entrance made out of elk antlers. Hanging from the centre of the arch was a large moose antler with "Welcome to Skyline, Pardner. Last of the Ol' West" painted across it. It was here, beneath the moose antler, that the nightly shoot-out was staged.

"Right on time," the master of ceremonies barked through the loud-speaker as a stagecoach parted the crowd in the intersection. Its wooden wheels clattered to a stop in front of the announcer, who was standing by the archway. Suddenly, two loud pistol reports startled the spectators. A man dressed in black, riding a slue-footed pinto, trotted up to the coach. A bandanna was drawn over his nose, and one eye was covered by a sinister black patch. There was an audible gasp as his pistol waved wildly in front of the tourists' faces.

"What's this!" exclaimed the announcer with melodramatic pretense.

"Oh, no, it's Black Bart! Quick, somebody get the sheriff!"

"Your money or your life," Tulip slurred through his bandanna to the coachman.

"My wife?" asked the bored driver. (He'd asked the same question every summer evening for the past three years.) "Sure, take my wife!"

"Not your wife, idiot!" the announcer burlesqued. "Your *life*!"

Actors playing the sheriff and his posse arrived. There was more shooting and overacting for the crowd, until Tulip finally ran out of blank bullets. A hangman's noose was thrown over the elk-antler archway.

"Wait a minute!" protested the announcer. "You can't just hang him. Not without a fair trial."

"All right, we'll give him a fair trial," said the sheriff, turning to the audience. "All those who think he's guilty, say aye." A number of the tourists responded. "All those who think he's not guilty, say aye." A few more answered. "Well," the sheriff said smugly. "The ayes have it! Guilty as charged!"

"Lynch him!" someone yelled from the direction of the Tumbleweed.

"I want a shoot-out with the sheriff," growled Tulip.

"What do you say, Sheriff? Do you want a shoot-out with this polecat?"

"I ain't scared of him. Cut him loose!" ordered the sheriff.

"Lynch him!" Earl yelled again as he, Jackson and the rest of their gang pushed through the crowd.

Buddy was surprised how smoothly it went. Fireweed collected the first two actors in his path. With one man under each arm, he slammed their heads together with such force that one collapsed to the ground unconscious. The other actor was dazed, and he tried to scramble away, but the Indian caught him by the collar and pulled him through the park. On the opposite side, on the street where Jackson had parked his camper, the women tied the actor's hands with his belt and locked him in the back of the truck. More of the gang arrived with more actors.

Buddy, for his part, grabbed hold of the bridle on Tulip's horse so the animal couldn't spook and accidentally lynch Black Bart. Simultaneously, Jackson eased up behind the show-boy sheriff and grabbed him, pinning the man's arms to his side. Earl took the microphone away from the stunned master of ceremonies, though not before the frightened announcer made a desperate plea for someone to get the sheriff. "The real sheriff!" he yelled, but no one responded, assuming it was part of the script.

"Ladies and gentlemen!" Earl tested the microphone. "Ladies and gentlemen, there's been a slight mixup tonight. You see, this ain't the *real* sheriff! Is you?" Jackson hauled the actor to the centre of the intersection where Earl jammed the mike in front of him. The actor was too scared to speak, and he shook his head.

"In fact," Earl continued, "he's actually in cahoots with Black Bart. Yeah, that's right, he's part of Bart's gang!" Jackson hustled the actor away to the waiting camper. *"We're* the real posse!"

"Daddy, Black Bart looks kinda scared," said a boy from Iowa, pointing at Tulip. The rope was still around the desperado's neck and trailing up over the arch. Only now Fireweed was anchoring the other end! The villain's one good eye was as round as a silver dollar.

"That's what you're supposed to think," explained the boy's father. "It's supposed to look real."

"All right, folks, now let's do this right. What's it going to be?"

"Lynch him!" yelled Jackson, coming back from the camper.

"There, it's unanimous!" Earl concluded before anyone else could respond. "Tulip Meeker, alias Black Bart, for crimes of disturbing the peace, stealing Buddy's firewood and generally being uglier than the south end of a northbound mule"—the audience laughed—"I hereby sentence you to hang by the neck! Do you have any last words?"

Buddy drew the bandanna from the bad man's mouth. "Get the sheriff!" Tulip cried. Again there was laughter.

"Gag him! There'll be no snivelling in the Ol' West." Again the bandanna was pulled over Tulip's mouth and tied taut.

There was a commotion in the back of the crowd as a rotund, frustrated little man tried to push his way through the cord of people. Some looked at him momentarily, judged him of little consequence and closed ranks. Again he tried, and again he was rebuffed.

Pulling out his .357 Magnum pistol, Sheriff Bow fired a live round into the air. "Now, get the hell out'a my way!" he commanded.

"Aha! The sheriff!" Earl waved dramatically. "And just in time! This, ladies and gentlemen, is Sheriff Samuel Bow, the *real* sheriff of Skyline!" There was a burst of applause; the new twist had the audience hooked.

Jackson stepped up beside Sheriff Bow and, like a great friendly bear, put an arm around Bow's shoulder. "Sam," he said under his breath, "I wouldn't stir up too much of a fuss. Tulip's pinto there might just spook and maybe Buddy couldn't hold his bridle. Know what I mean?"

Bow looked anxiously at Buddy and the rope with Tulip on one end and Fireweed on the other. Futilely he scanned the crowd for back-up.

"What do you want?" Bow asked nervously.

"Justice." Jackson grinned. "Justice . . . and a warm meal, maybe a hot woman. And, oh, if it ain't too much, a jug of that Wild Turkey. But that's all, I promise."

"Say, folks, this being Saturday night. . . ." Earl started playing again to the audience, drawing their attention away from Jackson and Bow. "I'm reminded of a story about two nuns who went out on a Saturday night to sow their wild oats."

Oh, shit! Buddy buried his face in his arm, laughing.

"Then they went to church on Sunday and prayed for a crop failure!"

"I'll throw your asses in jail!" Bow snapped furiously.

"Come on, Sheriff, loosen up. You ain't gonna spoil the show for these folks, are you?" Jackson cajoled Bow.

"Git that goddamn rope *off* him! Before someone gits hurt."

"And let Tulip go scot-free? Now that ain't justice, is it?" Jackson protested. " 'Sides, what are all these folks gonna think? We gotta give them some kind of a performance. Just look at them there, Sheriff, they's hungry for blood!" Jackson gave Bow a punctuating hug. "Say! I've got it." There was false revelation in his voice. "How about we take the rope off Tulip and *you* have a shoot-it-out with him!"

"I don't care what it takes," Bow fumed, exasperated, "just get that goddamn rope *off* him!"

"Hey, folks!" Earl said. "Because you're such a good bunch, we've got something special for you tonight. Skyline's very own Sheriff Bow thinks hanging's too good for this no-count Black Bart, so *he's* going to shoot it out! What do you say to that?"

There was loud approval.

"Unstring 'im, boys, and give 'im a gun," commanded Earl. Fireweed yanked the noose off Tulip and jerked him from his horse. A gun was jammed into the desperado's trembling hand, though the gag was left in his mouth. Jackson let go of the sheriff.

"OK, men. Now when I count to three, draw and commence firing. Ready? One!" Earl began.

Jackson watched the sheriff closely.

"Two!"

"Make it real, Sheriff," said Jackson.

"Three!" Earl yelled.

Either Bow had forgotten that he had real bullets in his pistol or he was simply planning to fire off a round in the air and his gun went off too soon. But a bullet tore through the archway, exploding antlers and showering Tulip with shattered bone fragments. Tulip was so happy to be alive, he fainted.

"Oh, my God!" Bow swore under his breath, his gun hand limp at his side. He stared with disbelief at the grapefruit-sized hole in the arch. He'd never witnessed the Magnum's power. Suddenly there was an outburst of applause. It brought him around, and slowly, like a rising crescent moon, a big grin swept across the sheriff's face. Holstering his pistol, he hitched up his pants, beaming. It had turned out all right after all. He smiled. Then he frowned, remembering Earl and Jackson. The microphone lay abandoned on the ground near Tulip, much to Bow's relief.

"Did you see the sheriff's face?" Melody gasped. To avoid capture, the gang had broken up. She and Buddy had ducked down an alley and were hiding behind two trash cans, holding their sides and laughing hysterically.

"And Tulip!" Buddy wheezed, winded from running and laughing. "Tulip never did put it together. Too bad he blacked out so soon. He might have had a heart attack had he seen how close he came to being on a slab at the morgue."

"Well, I think we put a wrench in their gears tonight!" Melody smiled, pleased with how the coup had gone.

"Naw, we just greased them, I'd say," Buddy said sarcastically. "Stoked more coal on their fire. Tomorrow, when word gets around that there was a near killing, there'll be *twice* as many people ogling the show!"

"I doubt that Tulip will make an appearance!"

"Well, there you are, at least we won something!" He smiled. Then Buddy peered around the trash can. Satisfied that they had escaped, he stood up. Faintly in the distance, he could hear the heavy thump of cowboy boots on Main Street's boardwalks. Cattle crossing a plank bridge, Buddy thought.

As they walked down a back street towards the laundry, Buddy was surprised to realize that Skyline in the summer was a real town! There were kids playing kick-the-can and couples sitting on front steps watching for the first lip of moon to rise above the peaks. There were crickets, the occasional dog barking and women humming through open windows while ironing their children's Sunday clothes. All he'd ever seen of Skyline in the summer was the Saturday-night side.

"You going to work at the laundry through the winter?" Buddy asked as they walked.

"You kidding? It's just a summer job. But I'm not sure what I'll do. The last three winters I went to music school in Utah, but I've graduated. I'll probably stay home in Idaho this winter and teach. I want to save up my money and travel."

"Yeah? Where you going to go?"

"Europe. Paris, London, probably Germany first. An old boy friend is on a mission for the church someplace in Germany. Maybe I'll look him up."

"Mission? You Mormon?" Buddy was surprised. "That why you went to school in Utah?"

"My father's bishop of the Driggs Tabernacle. Where else would they send me except Brigham Young University?" she asked.

"Breed 'em Young University! Yes, I've heard of it." It was an old joke he had heard from Earl.

"Breed 'em Young . . . hmm." Melody sounded slightly irritated, then smiled coquettishly. "Maybe that's why I'm attracted to younger men." Buddy clipped the heel of his right foot with the toe of his left and momentarily stumbled.

A block from the laundry, Buddy caught the not-unpleasant smell of scorched starch. The building was two-story, with a wooden staircase leading to the second-floor apartment. Buddy had been worrying about this moment for the past half hour. Should he suggest they sit on the steps and talk? Or maybe he should just say good-night and find Earl.

But she didn't give him the choice. Without breaking stride she started up the stairs. "Well," she said as she turned, "we can't stay out here. We're wanted criminals now."

The apartment looked like the inside of a gypsy wagon. Rugs, pillows for furniture and curtains for walls. What hard walls there were, were covered with posters from old movies. Monroe and Gable in *The Misfits*, sultry James Dean in *Giant*. Along one wall there were bookcases made of concrete blocks with boards painted black for shelving. There was a section of music books, some college texts and a few picture books of Europe. Buddy's eyes fell upon a stack of horse magazines.

"You like horses?" he asked.

"Sure. Don't you?"

"Better than walking, I guess, but just barely." Buddy picked up a thick volume of *The Book Of Mormon*.

Melody pointed to the book. "You're not anti-Mormon or something?"

Buddy felt her move close to him. "Tonight," he turned, smiling just inches from her face, "tonight I'd be a Hindu if that's what you wanted." Boldly he extended his hand to her hip, defined by the red dress.

"Relax, stud." She playfully pushed his hand away. Then she furrowed her brow as a teacher might to a delinquent student. "Don't want to start any bad habits, now, do we?"

She moved quickly away from him, turning on lights, turning off others. At the phonograph she spent some time looking through her records before finally putting one on. The music was strange and haunting, nothing like the shit-stomping songs Buddy felt comfortable with.

"It's flute music from the Andes," Melody said. "Can't you just see the mountains and the waterfalls? But of course, you probably see that kind of stuff every day."

"Bad habits?" Buddy asked. "What do you mean bad habits . . . like spreading social diseases?" He tried to sound like Earl, mature, informed. Unfortunately, except for the old *Playboy* magazine in the outhouse, Earl was Buddy's sole source of sex information, and most of that was what Buddy gleaned out of the cowboy's jokes.

"Bad habits"—she turned on him—"like trying to angle your way into a woman's undies. Shame on you!" she scolded him playfully. "You've got to learn to let a lady cream in her jeans! There's beer in the icebox. I'll be right back." Melody walked behind a curtain dividing off the bedroom.

Though his mouth was dry and sticky, Buddy didn't want any beer. He was confused enough; besides, he wanted his senses sharp, just in case. In the refrigerator he found a jar of orange juice and in the cupboard a glass, but his palms were wet and the glass slipped. He caught it just before it broke on the counter. Relax, stud, he counselled himself. He wanted to take his boots off, his feet ached from running, but that might be too forward, he thought. Maybe she's just a prick tease, a lot of Idaho girls are, he thought. He decided to leave his boots on.

Melody had changed from her red dress, and stood beside

the curtain in a full-length terry-cloth robe that betrayed little of her body except her long bare feet. Buddy noticed the belt was only loosely looped over itself. Suddenly his fear of coming on too fast eroded to panic. She was a college girl, and older than him; what was she going to expect? A knot formed in his stomach and drew tighter as she crossed the room, holding his eyes with hers.

She wrapped her arms around him, drawing him to her. Then she kissed him. Bewildered, he tried to kiss her back with equal boldness. His hand found its way under her robe and settled lightly on her hip. Her flesh was warm beneath the robe, soft and comfortable like tanned deerskin, and suddenly Buddy was self-consciously aware of every callus and rope burn on his hands.

Melody began unsnapping his shirt.

Buddy shifted, embarrassed. "Bony shoulders," he apologized. "It's a male trait in my family, all the men have bony shoulders."

"Everyone has something," she reassured him and slipped his shirt from his shoulders. Then she moved away and untied her robe, letting it fall to the floor. Turning in the subdued glow of a floor lamp, she posed like a model and drew her hand across her buttocks.

"No ass!" She laughed. It was small and muscular, just slightly concave on the sides. "That's my deformity, no ass."

Buddy could hear the noise from Solda's Grill a block away. It was the only place in Skyline that stayed open all night. Earl's truck was outside with Taylor passed out in the back, a note from Betty Sue sticking out of his hat brim. Buddy didn't need to read it, he knew what it said. "Call me," and then her number. Repair and reform. Buddy laughed. Well, she'd have a lot of work to do on Taylor.

Inside, Elder Earl's cannon voice volleyed above the jukebox. He was doing his hellfire and damnation on the evils of drink, one of his favourite sermons when he was drunk and the bars were closed. Buddy spotted Earl behind the counter waving a spatula in his hand like a sceptre or a crucifix or maybe a microphone. Occasionally he turned in mid-sermon to flip the pancakes sizzling on the hot grill behind him. Either the three pilgrims sitting on stools at the counter were caught in Earl's spell or, more likely, they were praying for food.

"Children!" Earl ranted. "Little children, wandering the streets, searching every rummy's puking face for the daddy stolen from them by that whore, hooch." Earl let his voice hang with grief. A woman in his small congregation gave a soft, weepy sigh. It was fuel upon Earl's fire. "And the women!" He started rolling again. "Destitute wives, doing slop jobs just to feed those poor little kiddies. Or maybe worse!" He waved the spatula, drawing Buddy's attention to the corner where Elsie was dancing the hoochie-coo alone in front of the jukebox. "Women flaunting themselves like brazen harlots at any cowboy with a dollar in his jeans!"

Elsie laughed, throwing back her shoulders and defiantly shaking her heavy breasts at Earl.

Fat Solda sat in a booth, reading the *National Enquirer* with intense interest for the latest details of a world gone weird. She spotted Buddy at the door and waved him over.

"I guess that was some show you put on at the lynching." Solda grinned. "Wish I could'a seen it. Your friend Fireweed's in jail for an alley fight with two Shoshone. And the rest of the R Lazy S crew left about an hour ago, talking about taking a chain saw to some billboards along the highway. I got a good power saw, so I said, 'Have at her!'"

"I see you've booked evening entertainment." Buddy nodded towards Elder Earl, who was crying and turning bacon simultaneously, his tears spattering and sizzling on the hot grill. Buddy suspected it was the smoke from the burning bacon rather than honest sentiment that brought tears to Earl's eyes. Still, his congregation was impressed.

"Look here, Buddy!" Solda held up the paper. "'Aliens impregnate Ontario woman.' You think they'll sue for custody? And where they gonna hold the court case? On Mars?" She shook her head at the dilemma, then looked at her watch. She groaned as she shifted her weight onto her legs. "Break's over."

Buddy stepped behind the counter and took the spatula away from Earl. "Come on, parson, it's jammie time."

There was a sincere protest from his flock.

"Hallelujah!" Earl raved. "The prodigal son has returned from the flesh pits! God." He sniffed. "You even smell of women!"

A mile out of town, a car accelerated behind them, its headlights blazing full beam. Suddenly the reflection of a red flashing light snapped across the mirrors and dashboard of Earl's pickup. Buddy eased off the gas pedal.

"Step on it!" Earl commanded from the passenger side. "We'll outrun the son of a bitch!"

"In this garbage can?" Buddy started laughing. "You're crazier than Johnny Nisbett!" Buddy slowed and pulled over to the side.

"Out of the truck! Hands on the hood, spread your feet!" Bow yelled, a flashlight in one hand, his .357 Magnum in the other.

"Sheriff, you almost shot one man tonight." Earl held onto the truck for balance as he came around. "I'd think your killer instincts would be satisfied for a while."

"Cut the crap. Spread 'em."

"Hey, look, Sheriff, nobody got hurt," Earl continued, sensing a slight advantage. "You're a fucking hero. Everyone's talking about how good you done. Hell, man, I just don't know what got into us, we was homicidal crazy, doped to the eyelids."

" 'Sides," Buddy cut in, fearing Earl would blow any edge they might have. "We're headed back to the ranch now. You've done your job and run us out of town!"

Bow was quiet for a moment; the idea sat well. Besides, he had already put one of the gang behind bars. It was courting trouble to get too many of them in the jail at once.

"All right, Buddy, one time only because you're local and your folks are friends of mine." He lowered the pistol.

"Want a snort?" Earl reached through the window and pulled out a pint of Southern Comfort from the glove box.

Bow looked at his watch in the headlights. "Four twenty-seven. That's off duty as far as I'm concerned." He reached for the bottle, unscrewed the lid and wiped the neck on his sleeve. "That sure was some show! Skyline ain't gonna forget it for a long time." He laughed and took a drink. "Would you've *really* hung him if I hadn't come along?" he finally asked.

Earl considered the question momentarily. "Naw, we was just gonna scare him."

Bow took a second pull from the bottle and passed it back. "Bull shit!"

Usually the road home seemed twice as long as the one going into town, but not tonight. The pavement shone like a silver ribbon under the moon's brilliance, and Buddy felt as if he were navigating a spaceship through a blue crystal solar system. His copilot was hunkered down in the corner, one foot against the dash, his hat pulled over his eyes to shield out the moon.

"I always figured I'd one day have a small spread of my own," Earl moaned. "With a wife and kids. But now look at me, all my money down the goddamn toilet!" Earl started to cry with maudlin self-pity.

Buddy was not sympathetic. It was a weekly ritual, bereaved penance. Still, tonight Earl was at a new low.

"It ain't even the same no more. Like Elsie, I could have *had* Elsie, she was so wet she was dripping on her shoes. But somehow I just wasn't up for it. You see the way she was dancing for me at Solda's? She was so hot she would'a screwed a fence post, and I couldn't get it up! Jesus H. Christ, I couldn't even get it up!"

Buddy nodded, but his mind was elsewhere. He'd finally had *it* ... sex. And it was nothing like Earl's jokes suggested. In fact, just the opposite. Not hot and heavy and borderline vulgar; rather his experience with Melody had been light and joyous and free of inhibitions. Melody. What a perfect name, even if it wasn't hers. Her body was like a musical instrument, a flute that sighed and moaned, whimpered, then wailed like the hard wind through the tops of the pine. He was clumsy, but she was patient and unabashed, drawing him back and forth between play and passion until they held no distinction.

At one point during their concert, he suddenly wanted to own her, just for himself. "I love you!" he'd blurted.

"No," she'd replied with a soft smile, "you love to fuck me. And I hope you *like* me a lot, because I *like* you a lot. But," she said, looking gently at him, "that's not I love you. I love you is a special prize to save."

"Ah, Christ!" Buddy hit the brakes and the truck skidded sideways down the gravel road. Taylor, in the back, slammed against the cab like a loose propane bottle. Earl was thrown forwards against the dash; his knee crushed his hat brim against his face.

"What in the holy hell you doing!" he yelled at Buddy.

Buddy pointed out the windshield. There, standing in the middle of the road, caught in their headlights, was a big bald-faced roan horse.

"Taylor forgot to close the fucking gate last night! The horses are out!"

"So? We'll get them tomorrow." Earl shrugged.

"Today *is* tomorrow!"

The two cowboys stumbled from the pickup, leaving both doors wide open.

"We ain't even got a halter," Earl complained.

"We can use our belts. If we wrangle them home now, we can sleep the rest of the day. Taylor's too drunk to ride, so he'll have to drive the truck back."

"At least let's wait till we can see. It'll be light in a while." They sat down on the gravel road and leaned against the front bumper.

"I'm getting too old for this shit!" Earl finally said. "Fifty-two years old and all I got to show for it is this ratty pickup and another hellacious hangover." He cradled his head in his hands. "You do all right last night?" he asked.

For a long time Buddy didn't answer. "I'm going to Europe," he said finally.

"Now?"

"No, smart ass. When I get enough money together. Maybe next spring."

The hues of dawn broadened until the cowboys could see the vague outline of the horses.

Earl wiped his eyes with the back of his hand and pulled himself to his feet. "Give me your hat." He took Buddy's Stetson off his head before the younger man could react, and began picking up pebbles and putting them into it.

"What's wrong with yours?" asked Buddy.

"What's wrong with mine?" Earl smirked. "It's *mine*, and yours ain't!" Shaking the hat like it was a bucket full of oats, he coaxed the roan closer until he could put a belt around the horse's neck. Buddy used the same trick to catch a sway-back paint standing off the road in the sagebrush. Both horses were kid-gentle, which suited the two cowboys fine. Neither man was in the mood for a rodeo.

Buddy swung easily onto his horse and took off at a lope, excited and expectant for the new day. Earl crawled slowly onto the roan. Grumbling about another Saturday night, he turned the animal in the direction of a distant horse bell. He listed to the right, his head slumped forward with his chin on his chest. The drooping roan cantilevered to the left, its head low and close to the ground. Both doors of the pickup were wide open.

CLOWNS

IT WAS THEIR LAST RODEO TOGETHER. FOR FOUR SEASONS BUDDY had been José's understudy, and now José wanted Buddy to take over the act so he could retire. But the only reason it had been José and Olé *that* long was because of José. He was the real rodeo clown. Buddy was just the rube in his routines and an alternative target for run-amuck bulls. No, the prospect of graduating to prime target wasn't a career ambition for Buddy. He'd quit when José did.

It began for Buddy as a weekend's diversion from staring at the walls of his dormitory room. One Saturday morning in the early fall, he'd driven west of Denver, and stopped by chance at the fairgrounds of a small ranching community where the local cattlemen's association was sponsoring a rodeo. Just as some families are musical and others have tennis and country clubs, Buddy was raised on rodeo. But unlike his dad or his grandpa Slim, Buddy was never much good on the broncs. His pain threshold was too low and his IQ too high, his grandfather teased. But as soon as Buddy saw José, he knew he'd found his niche in the sport—not to mention his escape from the tedium ad nauseum of Philosophy 101.

As Buddy drove out to pick up José that final morning, he remembered his first impressions of José the rodeo clown. There was José, dressed in a Bozo wig, red-striped referee's shirt and Levi's bloomers, loping across the rodeo arena towards a dazed bull rider who'd just been plowed through the dirt by an animal they called Saint Peter. Buddy was surprised by José's agility in spite of his baggy pants slapping against his scrawny legs like church chimes and his suspenders doing double duty to maintain propriety. On his way towards the cowboy, José bent over and scooped out of the dust the cowbell that had been attached to the bucking rigging.

"Hey, Hank!" he called to the rodeo announcer. "Know why they put bells on bucking bulls?"

While the announcer repeated the question for the folks in the far bleachers, José started helping the cowboy towards the safety of the chutes. Suddenly their escape was cut off by Saint Peter. The bull had circled around and was coming at them head-on like a derailed diesel engine. "You'll have to go it alone," said José as he cut away from the cowboy and started straight at Saint Peter, clanging the bucking bell and yelling with the fervour of a unrepentant heathen. It was apparent to Buddy that Saint Peter wasn't afraid of mere mortals, no matter how insane, and he just lowered his head to the business position and picked up the pace.

José came so close to the bull that even the jaded cowboys kneeling by the chutes jumped to their feet. But then, just before the collision, the clown cut sideways out of Saint Peter's path, drawing him away from the crippled cowboy. The foot race was on. José sprinted with adrenaline speed, but the bull was only a stride and a half behind. Kids scrambled back from the fence as the clown leapt for the top rail. José folded over the rail and flopped to the other side just as Saint Peter thundered past, spraying the audience with dirt. Quickly, José looked to see that the cowboy was safe. "Ain't you glad bulls can't climb fences," José muttered for the benefit of those just dusted by Saint Peter.

"Say, José!" boomed the announcer from the other side of the arena, "you never told us, Why *do* they put bells on bucking bulls?"

José had to think for a minute to remember the punch line. "To avoid traffic jams!"

"To avoid traffic jams? Why do bulls need bells to avoid traffic jams?"

"Because their horns don't honk!"

Buddy had learned early that bad jokes and bravado are the substance of rodeo clowns. Blending buffoonery and bravery and keeping the carnage to a minimum and the audience amused, those were the clown's jobs. Though they were not without rewards. For the cowboy who'd just been thrown to the earth by a ton of bull, or for the wide-eyed kid with his face pressed against the arena fence, the most important person in the rodeo was the clown.

Buddy turned off the highway onto a long dusty road leading out to José's ranch on the Platt River. He was looking forward to the rodeo, but he sure wasn't anxious for the inevitable confrontation with José. He knew José was going to use every trick he could to get Buddy to take over their routine when he finally hung up his suspenders. How ironic, Buddy thought, that now he was going to have to argue his way out of the business, after spending so much time convincing José to take him on as an apprentice.

"A college boy?" José said, hardly glancing at him when Buddy presented the idea. "You figure bucking bulls can read diplomas?"

"Even the Lone Ranger wasn't really alone," Buddy argued. He wouldn't take no for an answer. And he came back the following weekend, and the one after that; watching, learning. Then, on the third weekend, just before intermission, José got his foot stepped on.

"I don't suppose you got any clown duds?" he grumbled at Buddy as he limped to the chutes. Buddy smiled. He had already cleaned out a second-hand store of baggy, gawdy and garish clothes in anticipation.

"Git 'um on and I'll show you the ropes. 'Sides, the way you been hanging round, folks are starting to think you're my boy friend."

José scrutinized Buddy closely once he was dressed. "Olé! That's what we'll call you. It'll be 'José can you see by the dawn's early light' and 'Olé me down in the clover, roll me over.' But," he snapped, "git yourself another wig for next time. Orange is *my* colour—goes with my red eyes."

José was sitting with his dog on the front porch of the ranch house when Buddy drove in. José, a.k.a. Ben Riley when he was out of grease paint, was an archetypal cowboy. Tall, lean, weathered, with a horseshoer's hitch to his saunter and an

Alberta slouch to his hat. He was the stuff that Hollywood made movies about, only to cast the lead with rhinestone Redfords. But Ben didn't care, he wasn't interested in the big time. He was perfectly content to just be José and work the rural rodeos around his home range. Still, after four decades of baiting bulls and making a fool out of himself, and five and a half decades of hard cowboying, Ben had finally decided to put José out to pasture.

"Hey, Kemo Sabe!" He put his tattered suitcase in the back of the truck, then he went to the porch and returned with a giant inner tube. "When we get through today, you might as well take this stuff with you. I ain't got no more use for it."

"Ben, get it through that mass of scar tissue that you call a brain, I'm not taking over."

"We'll see." Ben smiled and got into the pickup.

An enclave of dusty pickups was already forming behind the bucking chutes at the rodeo grounds. Scattered around piles of saddles and bucking rigging, huddles of cowboys discussed the bulls and broncs they'd drawn. Buckle bunnies in tight jeans leaned seductively on fenders surveying the riders. Bruce Springsteen sang about cruising the mansions of glory on suicide machines against a background din of rodeo animals and handlers bashing about in the stock pens. It was the rhapsody of the New West, Buddy mused, jangled, jackhammer-driving rock, full of grit and glory, fuelling courage and illusions of immortality.

"Ah." Buddy nodded at the scene. "The narcissism of nihilism."

José erupted with laughter. "The narsissy of what? You trying to impress me, college man?"

Buddy thought for a moment. "Loosely translated"—he tried to sound professorial— "moths showing off before the flame."

José smiled. "That's a young man's game." Then he pointed to the other side of the chutes. "Let's land over there. Ain't so congested with narsissies." Buddy parked on the grass of the rodeo ground with his tailgate facing the arena's rail fence. He shut off the engine. José pushed in a tape of Hank Williams sagebrush-twanging about cheatin' hearts. Both men leaned back against the seat, staring out at the prairie running miles before the first tree.

"That sure don't look good." José pointed at a wall of black clouds forming against the eastern horizon. An ominous gust of wind off the pending storm swept up a boil of blinding arena dust. "Dust or mud, they're both just as dangerous as the other," José reflected. "Dust so thick that you don't see the animal that tramples. Or mud so deep that you can't git away even when you do see him coming."

Buddy decided to get it over with. "So why me?" he asked. "Why don't you just get one of those college-trained bullfighters to take over? You know there're a lot of schools around that give courses and scholarships in rodeo clowning."

"Too specialized for my tastes," José grumbled. "Nowadays they're all bullfighters, not ordinary clowns. And that's *all* they do, just work the bulls. They don't know squat from bootblack about entertaining audiences. For that, the sponsors got to hire a specialty act to come in with singing dogs and horses that can count higher than their owners. Nobody does both any more. But not you—you're country. You're a hick," he added with a great grin, "a born-and-bred rube."

Buddy was flattered. It was José's way of saying he thought Buddy was cut from his own weave of cloth. "Nope," Buddy said with determination. "When you hang up your suspenders, mine will be on the adjacent peg."

"We'll see," said José as he opened the door. He picked up the suitcase and walked around to the tailgate. Buddy joined him, and silently they began the precise task of making themselves look rag-bag ridiculous, and still be streamlined and fleet of foot.

José stripped to the waist and began wrapping his rib cage with an elastic bandage. He said it was for prevention, but Buddy suspected it was to keep the protruding points of previously broken ribs all working as a unit.

"The trick to staying healthy," mused José, "is knowing the animal and knowing what you can get away with. I can read an animal the way most folks read labels, and that's why I don't *ever* get hurt. Here," he said, pointing to his lower lumbar, "put your knee in my back there and try to straighten those vertebrae." There was an audible snap as the vertebrae momentarily aligned. José stretched and put on his Hawaiian shirt, then his Day-Glo leggings.

"That's some wardrobe," remarked a passing cowboy. "Looks like your mother dressed you in the dark!"

"You know," said José, leaning forward while tying his cleated track shoes, "they say a rodeo clown is a prime fool in a contest where *everyone* has a shot at the title. Maybe today will be *your* turn!" Then he smiled and accepted a pull on a soda bottle that wasn't pure soda. "Leastways I get to dress the part."

Rodeo clowns, Buddy realized, are the necessary splash of melodrama, giving perspective to the drama of the cowboys. Where the rodeo cowboy's dress is a clean-cut, stylish Stetson look, clowns are prairie punk. It's the attire of the anti-hero playing back up, and pickup, to the cowboys' heroics. The costume of the unwitting Charlie Chaplin, buffooning his way with deft finesse through fate's calamities.

Unwitting, Buddy thought. That's a good way to describe José and his routine. It was mainly impromptu, a mixture of broad-brush slapstick and a lot of split-second ad-libbing. They had developed a repertoire of a dozen skits and memorized a laundry list of punch lines, but, as Buddy knew from the ranch, working with livestock is too unpredictable to be routine. It was like being a barmaid in a logger's bar, he imagined. All you could do was react to the moment and hope you'd be around to collect a pay cheque when it was over.

"I remember once," José recalled, as he anchored his wig with bobby pins, "I used to do this stunt where I'd catch a bulldogging steer by the tail and let him pull me along until I'd got a good head of steam, then I'd do a flip in the air. But this one time I'd done my act and was walking away, figuring the steer was headed for the catch pen. All of a sudden, I looked around and there's the steer with his horn in my hip pocket. Well, I didn't know what to do, so I just pretended it was all part of the routine, and when I took off running, I started calling to the steer so people'd think I'd spent weeks training him to follow me."

Suddenly a scratched Johnny Cash record blared over the loud-speaker and a baritone voice called the riders to their mounts for the grand entrance. The grand entrance always amused Buddy. It was rodeo's equivalent of "Pomp and Circumstance," with a strange invocation called the cowboy's prayer. "And Lord, when we reach the pasture in the sky, may our entry fees be paid in full! Amen."

Hastily, José and Buddy gathered together the tools of their trade: the giant inner tube, the brooms and balls, the cardboard suitcase harbouring a scrawny rubber chicken, a dress and an oversized bra. From the top fence rail, Buddy paused, glancing momentarily at the pillar of rain clouds standing perpendicular behind the chutes. An anxious knot formed in his belly. Too late now, he thought, it's show time! It's José and Olé.

José set up his trap line for buckaroos—as he fondly called anyone shorter than his belt buckle. This entailed tying a rope securely to one end of a broom, then feeding the other end of the rope through the mesh fence separating viewer and viewed and letting it dangle there like a fat tempting worm in front of trout. "Now *don't* touch that!" José warned the kids on the other side of the fence.

"Say, Hank," he called, turning away from the fence. "Ya know my partner Olé? He's so dumb that when his sister asked him to name her twins, he named the girl Denise!"

"Why's that so dumb? That's a pretty name," replied the announcer.

"He named the boy Denephew!"

Turning back to the trap line, José found it full. "Let go of that, you buckaroos!" José growled and began a tug of war with the kids.

"Wow! Did you hear what that clown called me? A buckaroo!" A kid maybe six years old went scurrying excitedly back to his parents. Like a handshake from a politician or a smile from a beauty queen, a tug of war through the fence with the rodeo clown was a chance to share in his limelight, mottled as that might be. From that moment on, as far as the buckaroos were concerned, there were just two people in the arena, the clowns José and Olé.

The first event of the afternoon was the men's roping competition. Though it was a working event for José and Buddy, untying calves, corralling them, working in skits as time allowed, it was also a chance to loosen up the muscles and shake off the butterflies. They went through ten ropers and an equal number of jokes smoothly enough, but all at once the sky turned evil dark and split open, pouring with faucet force. The casual spectators raced for the beer garden or the parking lot, leaving only the true aficionados and the hard-core hands to continue the events.

It was rodeo at its rawest, stoic, Spartan roots—the way it was a hundred years ago, Buddy imagined. His instincts told him to find shelter. He looked at José.

"Why, you candy ass!" José laughed, the rain running down his face in rainbow-coloured streams from his make-up. "As long as there're contestants, we'll be here to tow 'em out of trouble."

Buddy looked at the faces of the cowboys behind the chutes. It was obvious that no one was going to show the white feather and quit.

"Insanity by association," he muttered to José.

"Well, *you* wanted the job." José grinned.

The next event was the Little Britches rodeo, kids riding spring calves. Few contestants showed, and those who did returned from their rides looking like the before side of a detergent commercial.

"Take care of my son!" an attractive mother in saddle-shined jeans called, smiling.

"She likes you." José nudged Buddy. "Take care of her kid and she'll warm your feet tonight. The real good lookers always want to go home with the clowns."

Buddy followed the calf out of the gate until the kid was about to be thrown, then he snatched him off the calf's back.

"Why'd you do that, mister? I could'a ridden him!" The kid started kicking Buddy. "Mom! That clown kept me from finishing!"

The mother eyed Buddy as if he were a convicted child molester, then said something unbecoming her beauty and disappeared behind the chutes.

"That lad's about the age I was when I started," reflected José as they set up the arena for the next event. "When my brother and I were youngsters on our folks' spread, we'd ride anything with hair! And of course, the highlight of our summer was entering the Little Britches, which eventually led to regular rodeoing and then into clowning."

Buddy once asked José what motivated him to put on grease paint and intentionally put himself in front of a muscled mass of meanness.

"Wages," he'd replied, then he laughed. "Course some say I'm just a natural born fool, anyway!"

Buddy suspected that the real reason was self- interest... therapy for the alter ego, exercising primeval needs for cheap thrills by flaunting oneself in fate's face. It was the fundamental attraction rodeo had for all participants — going beyond one's fears, and in an instant sorting through the calamity and coming up with a response that left you unharmed when the dust settled. Anyway, as José had often warned him, addictions don't need justification.

Because of the rain, there was no intermission. Jokes either misfired or were intentionally sabotaged by Hank, the announcer, who was anxious to get home. The bareback and saddle bronc events went fast. If a rider wasn't sitting on his mount by the time the last cowboy hit the mud, it was a no-show—no time, no money. Occasionally a horse would make a high, pile-driving plunge out of the gate, hit the ground with the force of a falling piano and then just stop, completely confounded by the mud. One cowboy demanded a re-ride. "Re-ride!" exclaimed a judge, pointing at the rain. "If you want re-rides, go to Madison Square Garden!"

The next horse out of the gate was a spinner, turning doughnuts in front of the chutes, sending cowboys scrambling up the rails in their stocking feet, their boots still stuck in the muck below. Then, suddenly, the horse lost its balance and started to fall onto its rider. Reading the animal, José was there just as the horse hit the mud. Catching the bucking rein, he pulled up the bronc's head, preventing him from rolling over on the cowboy. The rider scrambled under the bottom fence rail, and José hung onto the horse until he could get his legs beneath him and get up.

The ladies' events went smoother than the men's, in spite of the progressively degenerating weather. Then, about midway through the goat tying, José pointed to the next contestant, who was dressed in a fine lavender and lace cowgirl outfit. Every rodeo has a queen. Sometimes she comes out of the rodeo ranks and knows more about the sport than most cowboys. But this one, Buddy had a feeling, was picked by the town council for her congeniality and physical endowments, and she was obviously a neophyte to the rodeo scene. However, rural rodeos, Buddy had learned early from José, were no place for pretense.

"She's got her nose so high in the air"—José laughed—"she still hasn't noticed it's a sea of shit out here." Still, she somehow loped her horse across the arena without losing her hat and delicately dismounted—only then realizing what she'd gotten into. Timidly she minced towards the goat. But the goat, a veteran to the sport, stayed just out of her reach.

"I'll give her a hand," said José, and before Buddy could grab him, he entered the fray.

"Oh, shit!" Buddy exclaimed, expecting the worst. Just as he feared, the goat, the gal and the clown were suddenly intertwined in the goat's rope, and then they were mud wrestling. There was a great deal of flapping and flailing and José feeling up the rodeo queen before the woman and the goat broke free from him. Unfortunately, instead of accepting her plight with humour, the queen went berserk, slinging mud and foul language at José, the goat and even poor Olé.

"Well, I guess that's one looker that won't be keeping your feet warm tonight," Buddy teased. "But I do think she likes you." The queen was still shrieking at them—but from outside the arena fence.

The next event, the final event, was the clowns' main reason for existence—the bull riding. Always before, José had been the one to get in front of the bull and draw him out into the middle of the arena, while Buddy stayed on the side, ready to help the rider. But since this was Buddy's last day as a rodeo clown, he'd decided to try first-hand the terror of taking a bull on the nose.

"The main thing you got to do is pull the bull away from the chutes," José counselled Buddy, pleased at his interest, "because that's where most accidents happen. Mind you, when that gate opens, you got to have the jump on him and be ready to move, otherwise he'll nail you right in your tracks." Then José gave Buddy a hard, punctuating look. "But, damn it, son, if you don't stick around long enough to get the bull's attention right off, there's no use even being there! And the *only* sure way to get his interest is make yourself an attractive target—give him some hope of killing you!"

Buddy sucked in his breath. He knew that getting killed was very unlikely, but the clown's worst nightmare is the bull that doesn't lead—the one that gets away and throws his rider off the suicide side, twisting the bucking rope the cowboy has been hanging onto for balance into a death wrap around his hand. Then the rider's only release is for the side clown to lunge across the animal's back and jerk the loose end of the rope free.

"Don't be afraid to stay close to him," said José. "You've got a bull barrel out there to jump into if you get in trouble." He pointed to the middle of the arena and the fifty-gallon barrel, padded and open at both ends.

Buddy located himself in front of the chute. "Outside!" the rider yelled, and the gate swung open. The bull exploded at Buddy with the power of a full-throttle Harley in the hands of an angry biker. Damn, Buddy thought, what have I done? All his instincts screamed *run*, but he froze, probably more from fear than volition. Still, he held his ground for that instant it took to draw the bull at him. Then, thrusting his broom in the bull's face, Buddy headed for the open arena. Even soggy, the earth shook as the bull pounded behind him. But suddenly the animal swapped ends, trading head for heel, and took off in the opposite direction.

"Je-sus H!" Buddy swore at himself. "You've lost him!" Fortunately, José swooped in from the side, catching the bull's attention and leading him until the rider was thrown free.

While the cowboy ran for the safety of the chutes, José began taunting the bull.

"Get the inner tube," he yelled to Buddy.

Buddy ran to where the tube leaned against the fence, flopped it into the arena and waited for José to bring the bull in his direction. Just as the bull charged him, Buddy rolled the giant doughnut straight at him. The bull hit the tube with such force that for an instant it buckled into a bow, then flew high into the air. Again the bull charged. This time there was a bang louder than a clap of thunder, and a hissing sound like a punctured tractor tire. Startled, the bull jumped back a few steps as the tube propelled itself in psychotic circles through the arena mud. He attacked it again, but there was no use, the tube was dead. Then he spotted Buddy, a fully inflated, moving target. Again the foot race was on. Buddy dived for the barrel, standing on end, and was halfway into it when he realized José was already in there.

"Occupied," José wheezed, scrunched down in a fetal position to make room for Buddy. Buddy's face folded to the contour of José's track shoes, and his elbows jammed into José's eyes. He tucked in his legs just as the bull hit.

"Holy shit!" he yelled as they heaved end over end, then started spinning on their side like a carnival ride. Through a small opening between José's left knee and his right ear, Buddy caught glimpses of rain clouds, the chutes and all too often, a fierce eye and fiery nostril blowing steam into the barrel.

Then for a moment it was calm. José suddenly erupted with a wild maniacal laugh, the laugh of a kid in the front car of a roller coaster. It was contagious, and Buddy started, but then he felt José ease his head out his end of the barrel.

"Follow my lead," José ordered, rocking the barrel. "Eh, Toro!" José yelled. "Toro, *ven aquí!*" José quickly pulled back. *Boom!* came the clap of thunder, and again they were tumbling topsy-turvy. Twice more the bull punched the barrel, and they spun and rolled until Buddy felt sick to his stomach. Again José started to inch out.

"Stop it," Buddy yelled at him, "or by God, I'll puke all over you!"

"You candy ass." José laughed and pulled his head back in. Neither moved as they waited for the bull to lose interest.

"Man, how can you even think about giving this up?" José whispered.

"How can *you* give it up? It wouldn't be nearly so interesting if you weren't in here with me!"

Finally, José eased all the way out. Buddy followed, but he felt like an origami crane when he tried to straighten. Quietly they snuck close to the catch-pen gate before alerting the bull. The animal charged, the gate slammed shut and both clowns collapsed again with laughter.

The last bull of the day was a runner. Buddy had learned from experience that some animals spin, some fishtail—twisting their hind end like a wet towel in a locker-room fight—but this one was a sprinter. Buddy was slow on his takeoff, his cleats weighed down with snowshoe-sized clods of mud. The bull promptly outdistanced both Buddy and José. Luckily, the rider stayed with the animal and swung clear at the sound of the buzzer.

The contest was over. Buddy moved towards the bull, intending to draw him back to the corrals, but just as the bull turned, he slipped and unceremoniously went down. When he came upright, the bull's left hind leg was broken.

"Ah, he's not really hurt," Buddy heard an uneasy parent reassuring his concerned son. But Buddy knew better. The beast would be butchered by nightfall, and likely chilled then grilled next week in some service-club kitchen at another rodeo in another town. Unfortunately, he and José still had to get the animal out of the arena. To Buddy's astonishment, the bull made a three-legged charge at him. Slowly Buddy backed towards the catch pen while José brought up the rear, supporting the bull's bum leg by putting his shoulder on its hip and pushing each time the animal put pressure on the leg. It sure wasn't how Buddy had envisioned the end of José's and Olé's careers.

"Want a beer?" Buddy asked José as his pickup followed a family's station wagon through the lake that once was the parking lot.

"Might as well. Can't dance dressed like this."

There was a morose mood in the truck. On the radio, Willie Nelson warned mothers not to let their babies grow up to be cowboys—Buddy presumed, or rodeo clowns. He glanced at José. He looked pathetic with his wig plastered tight against his head by a mixture of grease paint, sweat and manure, hardly the profile of the survivor of a hundred bullfights and saviour of as many dazed cowboys. Are anti-heros, Buddy wondered, destined to anti-ends? No cheers, no jeers, just turned out to pasture after a rodeo that should have been stopped for rain in the first place.

At the intersection to the highway, they stopped behind the station wagon. One of the buckaroos in the back recognized José and waved. José waved back. More kids waved. José crossed his eyes, they crossed theirs. He made a comic face using his hands. They tried but couldn't, which broke them up into peals of laughter. The driver looked back, and Buddy noticed that he was the guy José dragged the horse off during the saddle bronc competition. The man gave José an appreciative wave before pulling onto the highway.

José sat quietly playing with the clasp on his suspenders. "You're not ready to be turned loose alone on the world," he said. "I've been thinking, maybe next season we should...."

TENN

"THERE'S NO REAL MYSTERY TO IT," BUDDY SAID, TALKING OVER his shoulder to the writer from *Sports Illustrated* as he undid the cinch and pulled the saddle off the back of the sweaty horse. Taking a terry-cloth towel from a stall peg, he began rubbing down the polo pony. "No mystery if all you're asking is how the tournament got started. But"—Buddy grinned, turning to face the reporter—"I suspect what you're *really* after is how did a refined sport like polo take root among this bunch of rowdy yahoos out here in the Rockies." Buddy nodded towards the cluster of men changing their jodhpurs and polo shirts for faded Levi's and western blue denim work shirts. There was a sharp contrast between them and another group of players getting dressed in clothes from Ralph Lauren and Brooks Brothers.

The journalist smiled sheepishly. "Well, maybe you're right." In fact, Buddy was exactly right. That was just the hook the writer's editor was after as soon as he heard about the polo tournament and the teams that would be playing in it from as far afield as Canada and Hawaii.

"Tenn," said Buddy without inflection. "Tennyson Fitzgerald Cabot the Third. He's your story, I was just a float in his parade."

"Is he here?" The reporter surveyed the players and polo fans milling around the perimeter of the stables and the field.

"Unfortunately, Tenn's dead."

"Hmm." The writer stared momentarily at his notebook. "Well, tell me, then, who *was* he?"

"Who was Tenn?" Buddy repeated the question, reflecting, organizing his thoughts. Buddy didn't know too much about Tenn's background except that he was raised on the fat side of Philadelphia society and had attended Princeton. When his widowed mother married a dude rancher in the Rockies, Tennyson quit school, shortened his name and came West with her. He'd told Buddy once that he hadn't been out West a week before he traded his Princeton letter sweater with a tiger insignia on the front for a Shoshone moose-skin jacket with an eagle beaded across the back. His oxfords went for a pair of high leather boots and a stake in a cowboy poker game.

Tenn, Buddy remembered, was a circus-come-to-town sort of guy. He was different from the other ranchers in the Skyline Valley. For one thing, his face lacked their hardpan, winter-wolf features. Instead, his countenance spread warmth like a driftwood campfire, and his lake-blue eyes seemed perpetually on the threshold of a joke. Maybe it was because Tenn was a cowboy by choice rather than necessity. Also, he was embarrassingly open rather than closed and taciturn, and you didn't have to know him very long to know him very well.

Tenn was a gentleman rancher. He was a gentleman foremost, and he made his living guest ranching gentlemen and gentlewomen. Men in blue Abercrombie and Fitch work shirts, with Swiss Army knives hanging off their smooth Bergdorf belts. Men who caught and released trout and donated large sums of money to wildlife foundations. And with them came gentlewomen. Ladies with languid eyes, wearing tan jodhpurs and orchid print blouses and soft lime-green sweaters drooping over their shoulders like bored cats. Sedate women, boarding-school women whose guarded and superlatively thick speech never flushed or faltered, except possibly when they were alone with Tenn, which, Buddy suspected, was more often than either Tenn or the ladies let on.

You could say Tenn was a peddler of dreams—with a special twist. He made them happen. His passion in life was participatory living rather than just fantasizing or watching. And as a result, a strange cult of esoteric characters gravitated to him. Probably, Buddy thought, because Tenn never judged. He offered unquestioning acceptance to anyone who shared his enthusiasm—no matter how obliquely it was expressed.

There were lesbian ranchers who listened to the thunder of Wagner amplified across their fields by speakers the size of hay bales. Counts stashed on cattle ranches with no-counts and remittance checks and strict orders not to return home lest they embarrass the family name further. There was this test-pilot pal of Tenn's from World War II, who flew the knife-narrow canyons between the mountains—sideways—and each Sunday he buzz bombed the ranch with a fresh copy of the *New York Times*. That is, until one morning when his hangover was as thick as the clouds shrouding the adjacent peaks and he took the top off a cottonwood beside the main lodge, and the FAA pulled his licence. There were stockbrokers turned stockbreeders, and a very expensive prostitute turned writer—except when her books weren't selling.

For the paying dudes, the attraction to the ranch, besides Tenn, was its opulent beauty. It was a self-contained village of maybe a dozen cabins huddled beneath skyscraper peaks that strained your neck and imagination to see their tops. Great hawk's head mountains lunging out over the valley, their cirques still filled with blue remnants of the last ice age.

The ranch's main lodge was a long and rambling log building with ivy on the outside walls and animal heads and western oil paintings decorating the interior ones. Original paintings by Russell and Remington of broncs bucking through campfires and wild-eyed cows being jerked off their feet by ropes guitar-string taut. Navajo blankets and cowhides covered the furniture and cascaded onto the polished wooden floors. They were hardwood floors that clunked with command beneath heavy cowboy boots, or sighed surreptitiously to the whisper of sheepskin slippers. But the western decor wasn't for the benefit of the dudes. It was authentic, and you didn't have to work at Tenn's very long to identify with at least one of the haywire situations depicted in the paintings. Like the time Tenn roped the moose calf and was chased home by its mother. Or the time he successfully blew up a stump with dynamite, though most of it flew through the large picture window of the main lodge.

Tenn's ranch was an institution that went far beyond accommodating guests. In one way, you could say it was a western finishing school. A place where generations of well-heeled Atlantic families sent their adolescent offspring to learn the realities of hard labour, of getting up each morning at five-thirty to an arctic cold cabin and a wrangle horse in a mean mood. This was standard curriculum; extracurricular activities included learning the proper language for earing down a bronc. And how to make Tenn's Meadow Dew Magic, a martini with a twist of pine needles instead of vermouth and grain alcohol instead of gin. Unfortunately, to the sponsoring parents' grief, many of Tenn's graduates would never again wear ties or dresses or attend DAR luncheons or ever, for that matter, feel comfortable in a building taller than one story. Also, whether by institutional ordination or just by luck, no one left the ranch a virgin.

Because of Tenn's divergent interests, his ranch was an intersection between two opposing cultures. It was a junction where the east-coast Main-line commuter train out of Bryn Mawr met the Powder River Grand Trunk railroad out of Rock Springs. Where maverick cowboys and Shoshone Indians herded dudes and horses with college football stars and sorority sweethearts. Mind you, the cultures didn't always mix, and occasionally a barn brawl would erupt, and sometimes pitchforks and shoeing knives were brandished—though seldom used. More often, however, it was debutantes in Levi's pitching hay and swearing with the zeal and regularity of a rodeo cowboy, and rodeo cowboys in boots, tuxedos and bewildered grins attending Philadelphia debutante parties.

Some say Tenn was a compulsive gambler. Buddy knew for a fact that Tenn would bet on anything from the weight of a trout before it was landed to Caribbean politics. But it wasn't a compulsion, he had too much class for that. Tenn did, however, acquire the ranch in a poker game with his mother. But that had more to do with the state's gambling tax versus inheritance tax. No, for Tenn, gambling was simply his way of giving an extra edge to events—putting a finer hone to the day's experiences.

As a consequence, one of the ranch's nightly diversions was the ritual of guests and crew congregating around the circular green-felt table at the lodge. Poker (considered the West's bastard sibling to the eastern games of bridge and backgammon) was the usual fare. Two kinds of poker were played at the ranch. There was "simply cards," a casual and cordial game that often degenerated into wild renegade versions like "Pick your nose in a coal mine," a game of grope-in-the-dark blind luck. Or "Sitting Bull," a game of pure bull-shit bluffing and blatant cheating. Fortunately, no money or property titles changed hands when "simply cards" was played.

"Big-boy poker," however, was different. When those guests and crew hardened to the drama of sweaty-palm, steely-brow poker sat down at Tenn's green-felt table, it was cards with significance. For one thing, the poker pots had substance, meaning that a wrangler's wages for a month or a week's worth of lodging for a guest and his family often lay in a frenzied heap of poker chips and tens and twenties.

Tenn played big-boy poker beneath a façade of rumpled nonchalance that masked the observant skills of a forensic psychiatrist. Instead of neurosis and psychosis, however, Tenn translated the subtle body signals into clubs and diamonds, straights and flushes. Little signs like a player's foot tapping nervously against the table leg or the heave of the dude's Adam's apple as he gulped down his drink, suddenly realizing that his cards didn't match his stake in the pot.

"This hand looks like a foot," Tenn would claim without conviction, while holding a winning hand. That was his opening gambit. Establish his credentials as a liar early, and then turn around and tell the truth the rest of the night. Still, you could never be sure with Tenn; he was also master of the backspin. "I've seen better hands on monkeys!" he'd grumble at his cards if he thought *you* thought he was telling the truth—all the while reeling you into betting against his straight flush. Buddy had a slight advantage in the big-boy games that allowed him to break even. He knew that Tenn bluffed worst when he had a winning poker hand and felt a twinge of guilt, and he lied best when he held a monkey's foot and needed to win. Still, losing to Tenn didn't really matter; you'd played in the majors. Like rope burns and saddle sores, it was a requisite exercise to being out West.

"You were going to tell me about Tenn and polo," the journalist interrupted Buddy's thoughts.

"Ah, yes, polo." Buddy smiled, hanging the towel on a wooden peg. He squatted and began unwrapping the protective bandages from the horse's leg. "Well, like most of Tenn's schemes, it began with a bet."

The writer looked dubiously at him.

"No, it's true, I was there when he made it. You see, Tenn and I had gone to town one rainy afternoon to pick up some horse feed and block salt, and we'd stopped at the Silver Dollar Bar on our way home. Harl Gibbons, another dude rancher with a spread directly across the valley from Tenn's, was there with some of his guests. And as the afternoon wore on, and their conversation wandered around through a forest of gin and tonics, Tenn and Harl hit upon the subject of polo—a topic neither of them knew too much about, except that it was the sport of sultans and both were feeling regal that day. Well, one half-cooked idea led to another that was even less baked, and before long a bet of considerable size was placed on the outcome of a match between their respective ranches, winner take all, rules to be decided at a later date.

"I didn't think much about it until a few days later when Tenn showed up at the bunkhouse with half a dozen mallets, an equal number of construction hard hats (for polo helmets) and a couple of softballs. Almost as an afterthought, Tenn pulled out a copy of *Polo, The Official Rules.*

"I remember how we studied the book's pictures, imagining ourselves locked in thundering ride offs and driving the ball through the goal posts to glory and the charms of an impressionable dude girl. No one bothered to actually *read* the rules. Besides, we figured there couldn't be that much to it— hit the ball, ride like hell, hit the ball and collect our winnings at the end of the match." Buddy laughed and shook his head.

"So Tenn began marking out a field three hundred yards

long by two hundred yards wide, there in front of the fish pond's embankment. Reasoning, I guess, that the slope of the embankment hill would make a good amphitheatre for the spectators plus a natural deterrent for runaways. Then we spent the next two weeks picking rocks, pulling sagebrush out by its roots packing the holes with dirt and grass seed and then compacting the field with a stoneboat and roller.

"There were four of us on that first team." He stopped undoing the horse's legging wraps and looked at the writer. "Besides Tenn and myself, there was a guy named Mike and a lady by the name of Tess. Mike came to the ranch from back East, but in spite of his New Jersey accent and a choirboy innocent face, he was a hell of a cowboy. And Tess was a riding instructor at one of those elite eastern girls' schools that crank out Olympic equestrian competitors with singular regularity." Buddy smiled. "She was really something! Had beautiful Egyptian skin, haunting dark eyes and the corral manner of a Marine drill sergeant. As I remember, she could make horses and wranglers either swoon or tremble, depending on her mood."

Buddy rolled up all the leg wrappings and moved to the horse's hind feet. "Our first task was picking our polo ponies. And from the outset, it was obvious that our inventory was going to be limited to horses that were either dude broke or half broke. Which is to say that they were either so docile they'd hardly budge from the corral or so wild they were climbing the corral fences to escape. Mind you"—Buddy smirked—"our criteria were equally wide. If you could swing a mallet and the horse didn't buck, it had polo potential.

"We then weeded the thirty or so potential mounts down to just six. Unfortunately, we'd also had to lower our standard to simply horses that didn't buck as hard as the others. And God, what a collection." He shook his head. "Of the six, there were two who looked moderately like polo ponies, if you squinted from a distance and used a lot of imagination. Unfortunately, they were both brain dead. We also had two short, stubby-legged horses who were real bulldogs in a ride off, but they were slow as dachshunds. The fifth animal was a horse named Mohammed, a strong, long-legged bay, fast and powerful in a ride off. Also he looked like a polo horse, loved contact and had a flat, even stride that was smooth as a gazelle's at a full gallop. His only problem was that full gallop was his *only* speed—unless you included completely out of control!

"Then there was Tenn's pet horse, Dexter. He was this purebred quarter-horse stallion who periodically broke down every fence on the ranch and bred every mare in a ten-mile radius. Tenn had won him off Farren Walters in a bet, as usual. 'Fair and square,' Tenn used to say. Course Farren claimed that he was glad to get rid of Dexter because of the horse's hormone problem, so he simply let Tenn win." Buddy chuckled. "But the real problem wasn't fixing fences—you, see, Dexter had this embarrassing habit of trying to mount any mare regardless of where she was standing or the immediate proximity of onlookers.

"Still, to be honest with you, in the final analysis it really didn't matter much how suited our horses were for polo—we still had only six and we needed at least eight." Buddy finished with the horse's leggings, then nodded to the journalist to follow him as he led the animal out to a large open pasture. There, Buddy threw the tie end of the halter rope around the horse's neck while he removed the halter, then he turned him loose. "You see," he said, leaning on the gate, watching the horse roll in the dirt, "with four players, we didn't have enough horses to rotate onto a fresh mount after each chukker. Still the other side was, we didn't have much choice, either, given the rank condition of our inventory. But we talked about it and we decided that we'd just have to beat Harl's team with sheer skill instead."

"That first practice was polo by Braille! We were like blind people in bumper cars the way we were crashing into each other!" Buddy frowned. "There were horses rocketing every which way, and riders clinging to their necks with one arm and flailing their mallets in the air with the other. Of course, since no one had read the rules, we were continually broadsiding each other. And it was only by trial and error that we realized everyone had to play right-handed so two opposing riders could pass on either side of the ball without a head-on. Mind you, there was no shortage of hard pragmatic lessons learned that day." Buddy snorted. "For example, it was only after a couple of real life-threatening accidents that we saw the importance of keeping an uncontrolled mallet away from the feet of a horse going full throttle."

He turned to the writer, shaking his head. "You know, there's nothing in the world so rude as having your horse suddenly cut out from under you. And nothing ahead of you but wide open spaces and an inevitable collision with the ground. And not only are you being rocketed into the dirt with the same momentum that only seconds before carried you heroically towards the goal and glory. Your horse is tumbling head over hooves right behind you!"

Buddy laughed. "It was only *after* our first practice, while we were laid up, nursing our wounds, that we finally got around to studying the rules. Everyone was pretty depressed. We didn't entertain visions of honour on the playing field any more. By then we were just praying that we wouldn't look like damn fools!

"But I will say, nothing teaches as well as pain," Buddy added, "and our injuries did put a new edge on subsequent practices. During those first few weeks we worked first on just hitting the ball. Off-side shots at a walk first, then a lope, then a gallop—or in Mohammed's case, hell-bent for leather! But eventually we got to the point where we were trying on-side shots and even neck shots.

"The next step was to start playing like a team. As you probably know, the key to playing polo, like hockey, is passing on the run, not to where your teammate is but to where he's going—leaving the ball far enough ahead of him so that he has time to set up his swing. We even got to the point where we could execute a few primitive plays—as long as we didn't have an opponent there to break up the dynamics of our passing and posturing. But you know, it was interesting, even the horses improved and seemed to enjoy the contact of ride offs, once we figured out that you weren't supposed to intersect another rider at a right angle. Mohammed calmed down some, and most of the time you could count on setting up at least a couple of shots each period before he lost control. And even Dexter seemed to have put his biological drives in park.

Buddy pushed himself away from the gate, suddenly realizing that the journalist had long since stopped taking notes. "But this isn't what you wanted for your story. I guess to answer your question, polo became westernized with a bet and a lot of pain."

"Wait a minute," the writer protested. "You can't leave me hanging. What about the game? I assume you played one. Who won?"

Buddy was surprised. "Well," he said reluctantly, "if you're really set on the gory details, let's at least get out of the sun." He led the way to the shady side of the paddock and sat down on a hay bale.

"The day of the match was a beautiful Sunday afternoon in August. Word about the game must have circulated all around the valley because there was quite a crowd of ranch guests, neighbours and even some outside tourists. Harl's ponies had arrived earlier that morning in a liner truck—ten of them! A rotation and two spares, which they weren't about to lend to us! But the worse part was, they looked like polo ponies, not glorified wrangle horses. Hell, we just hoped that our mounts looked like wrangle horses and not just glorified rodeo broncs! Still, I must say that our modest mounts bore only vague similarities to those sagebrush wild mustangs who'd two months before climbed fence rails whenever the ball came at them." Buddy grinned. "And thanks to Tess, they were all powdered and preened, and their tails back knotted so they wouldn't get tangled in our mallets. She'd even braided their manes with little ribbons knotting off the ends. Mind you, *we* were hardly recognizable ourselves. Clean white polo shirts, jodhpurs instead of Levi's, real polo helmets instead of hard hats and English riding boots instead of shit stompers. In fact, once Tess finished plaiting our ponies, she'd turned her shears on us and pretty soon we were looking like regular Ivy Leaguers. I will admit that even though we were strutting around like matadors, we were all secretly scared to death.

"You know, to this very day, I still think if Conrad had come down to the polo grounds with the rest of us, Tenn might have got away with it."

"Conrad?" the journalist asked.

"Conrad Benton. He was the son of a wealthy industrialist who owned the ranch down the road from Tenn's. Anyway, like I said, instead of slipping in with the rest of our team, he arrived late. And unfortunately, not only was he riding this big beautiful chestnut horse, he got there just as Tenn and Harl were counting out the bet money. There was *hired gun* written all over Conrad, sitting on that thoroughbred like he was fresh off the Cornell polo team—which, in fact, he was.

" 'You wouldn't try to sneak a ringer in on us, would you, Tenn?' Harl accused, drawing back his half of the wager. Tenn looked guilty as hell and nodded to Benton that they'd been caught. So Conrad tied his chestnut to the hitching rail and joined the rest of the spectators on the hill. As you can imagine"—Buddy smirked—"there was some hard rail leaning and horizon staring before Tenn and Harl began counting out their halves of the bet again. But finally the wad was given to the umpire to hold.

"It's my memory that the opening chukker was slow, each team feeling out the other, measuring each other's horses and horsemanship to find the animal afraid of the ride off or the rider who'd look up to see where he was going instead of concentrating on the ball. Still, we each muddled through to a goal apiece, though they were both pretty lacklustre. Unfortunately, however, by the end of the period the differences between our teams were beginning to show."

"In what way?"

"For one thing, while we had the advantage of practice, in that we could hit the ball with some regularity and they missed a lot of shots—they had the horses. And though our sturdy stock were solid as tanks in a ride off, they were simply being outrun.

"And sure enough, the second period turned into a predictable disaster and the score jumped to three to one against us.

" 'Doesn't look good!' I recall Tenn groaning, loud enough for everyone to hear, as he dismounted by the keg of beer separating the two teams.

" 'What's wrong, Tenn?' Harl asked, 'not trying to duck out of the bet, are you?'

"Well, Tenn just stared for a long time at his boots, not saying a thing. 'It was a thought,' he said to Harl, 'but now that I think about it, I believe we're starting to get the feel of this game.' Again he studied the dust on the toes of his boots. 'Want to raise the bet, say, double it?'

"Harl's hand was out to Tenn like a lightning strike. Unfortunately, I sure didn't share Tenn's intuitions. By my assessment, not only were we behind by two goals with half the game over, but we were out there on Ford station wagons pitted against Porsches—all of which just confirmed a long-held suspicion that betting, for Tenn, was an object in itself and had nothing to do with the subject of the bet or even its outcome.

"Anyway, we changed our strategy early in the third chukker. And we began passing and finessing the ball between us, back and forth across the field like a hockey line, all the while saving our horses by avoiding the hard ride offs and long pursuits. The technique worked well enough for us to pick up a legitimate goal, but soon Harl's boys adjusted to us and again we were forced to play defensively. Everyone started getting pretty frustrated, and it wasn't long before tempers began to flare and flying elbows and foul shots dominated the balance of the period.

"Now you got to picture this," Buddy said to the writer. "There we were between the third and final period, behind by one goal and needing two to win. Well, it was bedlam at the hitching rail. Saddles were being whipped off one horse and slapped onto another with a mania that comes with adrenaline and high stakes. Everyone was yelling at each other and no one paying the slightest bit of attention. I think Tenn was counting on the confusion.

"Luck seemed to turn in our favour with the first throw-in of the chukker. Tess was able to cut through the congestion and pick up the ball with a beautiful neck shot. She passed it perfectly down the field, right ahead of Mike, who was riding Dexter. Everyone on Harl's team was so startled by the shot that no one challenged Mike, and he fired the ball directly towards their goal. Still, it seemed rather hopeless, since Harl was in a good position to deflect the shot from going in. But, as fate would have it, Harl's mare was in heat—and upwind!

And just as Harl was in midswing with his mallet, Dexter caught her scent and tried to mount Harl's mare on the fly! Natually, she spooked and fled in the opposite direction, with Dexter in hot pursuit, Harl hanging on her neck, and the ball untouched just yards from the goal. Well, we all took off hell-bent for leather down the field towards the lifeless ball.

"I can't say that the game was a sport of gentlemen by then, more like a free-for-all of Kazakhstan tribesmen!" Buddy chuckled. "Everyone was clubbing the stuffings out of each other, swearing, throwing punches and all. But finally, the ball dribbled out of the melee (more from fatigue than force, I suspect) and rolled between the goal posts. The score was tied. Harl protested Dexter's attack, but there were so many infractions on both sides that the umpire decided to forget the whole scene.

"I thought lady luck was still smiling on us when Mohammed and I were given an out-of-bounds shot from our end of the field. However, with the excitement of the last goal, Mohammed was right on the edge of losing control completely. And it was obvious to me that he wasn't going to stand for a stationary shot, so, swinging him in a wide circle, I lined up the horse, the ball and the distant goal and just let Mohammed have his head—praying that he'd run in a straight line.

"God." Buddy sighed with a twinkle of nostalgia in his eyes. "To the day I die, I'll never forget the feeling of that mallet as it came against the ball. *Wumph!* He swung his right arm as though making the shot. For that incredible instant when the shaft arched backwards against the ball's inertia, I could feel the full power of the charging horse surge right up through my arm. And that ball took off down the field like it had been shot from a rifle!"

"Unfortunately"—Buddy sighed again—"for reasons known only to Mohammed, that's where play stopped for us that day. Instead of following the ball, he veered off line and slammed broadside into an opposing player! And even though the guy and his horse went down, Mohammed wasn't even staggered by the impact. He vaulted over both of them and charged up the embankment of the fish pond, scattering spectators out of the way like they were loose chickens. Thank God there was a freshly plowed hay field adjacent to the pond. After cutting a couple dozen roundhouse circles around it, with Mohammed's head sucked hard against my knee and his neck bent in a tight comma, he finally slowed down enough for me to bail off. I guess the infraction was just too blatant to be ignored by the umpire, and Mohammed and I were thrown out of the game for irresponsible conduct"—Buddy frowned—"as if I'd had any part in the matter."

"Anyway, I was feeling pretty discouraged there on the sidelines. And I suspected that it was just a matter of time before one of Harl's men broke loose and made the winning goal.

"But suddenly, with less than a minute left in the game, I realized what Tenn was up to. You see, in the confusion between chukkers, Tenn had thrown his saddle on Conrad's thoroughbred. Well, when he uncorked that horse of Conrad's, he was in there and scooped up the ball just as easily as can be. I figured Harl's boys would become suspicious when two of them tried to sandwich him between them and Tenn's horse lined out like a greyhound, leaving them in his dust. But I guess they were too startled to notice. Of course, Tenn was on the ball before it stopped rolling from his first shot. And it was just like we'd originally dreamed it would be, hit the ball, ride like hell, hit the ball, ride like hell. Three solid shots put the ball once again down by Harl's goal. Harl's mare must have still had bad memories of Dexter's charge, because she spun so quickly to get out of there, she almost dumped Harl on the ground. Tenn made the winning goal just as the closing gun fired.

"Tenn didn't even slow down, headed straight for the barn with the rest of us close behind. And of course, we immediately stripped our saddles off the horses and turned them out to pasture with the rest of the herd, where they promptly rolled in the dust and hid any evidence of foul play.

"Tenn threw one hell of a party at the ranch that evening, as best I recall. And between polo being the main subject of conversation and Tenn's Meadow Dew Magic the main fuel for derring-do, it wasn't very long before another bet was made for a return match the following summer.

"It wasn't until a few days after the game that Tenn mentioned the game to me: 'Can you imagine Harl accusing me of bringing in a ringer? As if we couldn't beat them fair and square.' Then I remember him smiling this wide, Cheshire cat grin 'It never was the rider I wanted, it was his horse, all along! Conrad just brought him down to the field for me.'"

The man from *Sports Illustrated* was holding his sides with one hand and wiping the tears from his eyes with the back of the other.

"And that," Buddy said, smiling with amusement at the writer's amusement, "that was the beginning of the Tournament of Tenns." He watched a man approach them from a horse truck parked at the end of the paddock. Buddy rose to his feet. "I don't know if you have a story, but it's all true."

"Oh, there's a story there." The writer stood and nodded reassuringly.

"I should add that over the next few years, the quality of horseflesh improved considerably around the valley. And the size of the wager increased significantly beyond the annual rate of inflation."

The tall man Buddy had been watching came up to them. He was the captain of the Vancouver polo team. "The trucks are loaded, so we'll have to be going," he said. Then he reached into the inside pocket of his sports jacket and drew out a fat envelope, which he gave to Buddy.

"See you next year?" Buddy asked, shaking his hand.

"You can bet on it." The man grinned.

COLLARING ABDUL

"BUDDY, GET SET BACK THERE. WE'RE COMING UP ON THE caribou." The pilot's voice was calm and level through the helicopter's headphones—a welcome relief for Buddy from the pervasive bark of the rotor blades overhead and his heart pounding in cadence against his rib cage.

Buddy looked anxiously across the seat at Marc and his grip on the safety line that ran to Buddy's chest harness. Marc flashed that damned irrepressible ain't-this-fun grin and gave the line a reassuring tug.

"Take a loop around your neck," Buddy yelled at Marc, forgetting that they were both wearing voice-activated microphones. "That way, if I fall out, you'll be right behind to keep me company!" It was a dumb thing to say, but Buddy wanted to emphasize to Marc that it was him on the end of the safety line, and not some errant steer on a Saskatchewan farm. Marc just kept grinning.

Turning to the open doorway, Buddy eased out to the lip of the seat, fighting back the nausea and trying to ignore the chaos outside the machine as they raced just yards above the muskeg. Placing one foot on the skid and the other on the step of the helicopter's forward strut, he settled into a shooting position, using his front leg to support the weight of the net gun.

Buddy wasn't sure what to expect. It was their first capture attempt with the net gun and the helicopter. All the caribou they'd caught and radio collared before were tranquillized from the ground. But the endorphin drug they'd used was too dangerous for animal and man—though Buddy still wondered just how safe this new approach would prove. The capture part of the project was the trickiest. But once the radio collar was secured to an animal, it transmitted a signal the team could monitor from the air without ever again entering into the animal's life.

There were four of them on the team. Greg, the pilot of the Bell 206 helicopter, was a great bear of a man with a rugby physique and a gift for flying the machine with the finesse of a flute player. Delicately feathering the stick between thumb and forefinger of his great paws, he'd inch the 206 through narrow canyons whose walls were sometimes only a couple feet from the tips of the blades.

Donald, the project's biologist, sat in the front of the helicopter beside Greg. He was a tall man with thick, cocker-spaniel hair and a meat-and-potatoes approach to biology. Donald had designed the project, and its elegance was its just-the-facts-ma'am simplicity—base-line studies of what was where and when, leaving the whys for the academicians and politicians to argue over. Buddy thought Donald had a very balanced perspective—for a scientist. "I'm going to biologize," he'd say, headed for the base camp outhouse with a roll of toilet paper in one hand and a folder of caribou data sheets in the other.

And then there was Marc. When he wasn't holding Buddy's safety line, he flew the fixed-wing airplane used for the monitoring flights. Once a month in a Cessna 185, Marc and Donald (and sometimes Buddy when his stomach could take it) combed the mountains and plateaus around the Spatsizi wilderness in northern British Columbia, counting caribou and fixing their locations. Marc was a lanky man who moved with the confident shuffle of a forty-points-per-game basketball player. He had a prairie-innocent face, boy-scout, at-your-service eyes that were never bored or boring and a river otter's sense of humour. Moreover, Marc was a man fulfilled. His sole ambition since he was fifteen was to be just exactly what he had become, a bush pilot.

Buddy felt like his contribution to the team wasn't nearly so interesting. He was the tin-cup rattler. Which meant that once a year, dressed in a Brooks Brothers three-piece suit and

Hermès tie, he would hit the offices of the private foundations, corporations and government bureaucrats, rattling the cup for funding. Fortunately, because the project was designed to focus on the fundamental questions and it had lots of high-tech gadgets and ecological sex-appeal, it sold itself. Also, Buddy had two assets that qualified him for his task. The first was a simple observation of Slim's, "Folks's just folks." Consequently, power, wealth, even pedigree had no more meaning to Buddy than a person's height or eye colour. His second attribute was a history of "academic hoop jumping," as he called his college experience, and he had acquired a couple degrees in zoology to prove his pain.

In a sense, it had been a linear path from Buddy's adolescence on the family ranch in Wyoming to the helicopter seat in northern Canada. He had been sent to university with specific orders from Slim to "get education and we'll beat those bastards at their own game." "Those bastards" were, in Slim's eyes, the government civil servants who were reducing the wilderness that once enveloped their ranch to public parks and leave-strips between clear cuts. It was at college, in his biology class, that Buddy met Janet. She had olive skin, daisy-fresh eyes and a Husky's love of being outdoors. She was from the East and knew the first time she saw the Rockies that she couldn't live anywhere else but the mountains. They were married after graduation and returned to Buddy's family in Wyoming. But it was too late. Buddy realized that the managers had already irreversibly changed the land and its wildlife.

He never told Slim or Casey outright why he wouldn't eventually take over the ranch's operation. But he saw that the wilderness of his childhood had been turned, by slow, incremental measures, into a glorified petting zoo. For one thing, the elk herds were being fed in the winter like cattle. And because they were a game species, a management decision had been made to maintain their populations at an unnaturally high level. That in turn led to overgrazing, and the displacement of the bighorn. The government responded to the overgrazing problem with a mass slaughter of nearly half the elk herd to bring their numbers in line with the carrying capacity of the land. But then three consecutively hard winters of deep snow and extreme cold hit, and the remaining population crashed. Within thirty years following the first management decision, the once great elk herds of the Skyline Valley were on the verge of collapsing.

The wolves had been systematically hunted to extinction by the fish and wildlife department because they competed with man for the elk. And, while the bounty hunters were at it, the government had decided, for the same reason, to have them kill off the big cats, the cougars and lynx. Buddy and Janet wanted elk that were afraid of man and wolves and cougars for their children to fear. They moved to northern British Columbia.

"Feed me line." Buddy rocked against the harness, feeling its pressure upon his chest. Cautiously he leaned outside the machine with the net gun, testing the effects of the wind and the rotor down wash. "That's about right. But pull up fast if we bank inside, or else I'll be plowing muskeg with my face."

"Could be an improvement," Marc teased.

"For me or the muskeg?"

"Okay, here we go," Greg cut in. "Hang onto your rosaries!" There was a ring of excitement in the pilot's voice. "Don't shoot us out of the air!"

The ground below Buddy began to accelerate. The muskeg and willow lost distinction from the puddles of marsh water as everything melted into a lime-green blur. Overhead, the foreboding grey shadow of the blades distorted the sky. His stomach heaved and he had to focus for a moment on the mountains along the far edge of the great meadow. The farther out Buddy leaned, the louder the rotor wash thundered in his head and the harder the wind tore at his earphones. Then, suddenly, the caribou was there, clear and distinct against the moving background. Reaching with long racehorse strides, its paddle feet splayed the spring-soft marsh grass, sending fans of water ahead, leaving deep imprints behind. Buddy was awed by the bull's grace and power until suddenly he focussed on something else. The antlers—even in velvet—were huge!

Buddy waited until the caribou was just slightly ahead of the skid before squeezing the trigger. The inside of the helicopter resonated with the explosion. The recoil drove Buddy's elbow hard against the door frame; his hand went numb. But the net opened like a magnificent red butterfly swooping above the caribou, wrapping its wings towards the moving animal.

"That's one!" he yelled, pulling back into the machine. But suddenly, to his astonishment, the trailing edge of the net snagged on an antler, and instead of collecting around the animal the way the manual claimed it would, it flared in front of him.

"Step into it!" Buddy coaxed, but the net closed too soon and dangled like a twisted rope off the bull's rack. The caribou spooked sideways and began fighting the net as he would an attacking wolf, lunging and swinging his antlers close to the ground—serving only to ensnare the nylon mesh even more around his rack.

Greg landed the helicopter fast and hard. They'd have to try catching the caribou on foot. Marc and Buddy swung out to the right, Donald and Greg to the left, trying to corral the bull between them. But it was no use. The net had twisted into a tight bundle around the caribou's antlers, and didn't slow him in the least. After half an hour of chasing and crashing through the buck brush, they realized they'd have to return to the helicopter and use a second net. Precious minutes were spent strapping the new net bucket onto the gun and sliding the greased weights down each barrel. By the time they were airborne again, the caribou and their first net had disappeared from the meadow. Greg lifted the helicopter vertically, like an elevator, and systematically began searching the forest, moving higher up the ridges with each pass.

"Eleven o'clock, near that pine snag." Greg pointed to the south. "Is that the one you want?"

"Is he wearing a Day-Glo turban?" Marc asked.

"The very one." Greg laughed. "But we can't get him in there. I'll have to move him away from the trees." Finally Buddy saw the bull in the heavy timber at the base of a rock ridge. He was snaking easily through the trees and cliff boulders, apparently unhampered by the net. Greg slowed the helicopter and, using the wind off the rotors, began gently herding the bull towards the open meadow.

"The ultimate ballet," Marc said as Greg swung the machine smoothly from side to side, finessing the caribou out of the heavy forest. "Peter Pan without strings."

Finally the bull abandoned the forest and began trotting down a wide, shallow stream separating the timber from the meadow flats.

"Buddy, I'll set you up just as he climbs the bank," Greg said.

"Let me out a little more," Buddy called to Marc. "I took a hard hit on the door jamb last time." Then, remembering the force of the wind upon his headset, he pulled it off and pitched it on the seat behind him.

"Okay, pilgrims, it's rosary time!" Greg said.

Again Buddy moved onto the lip of the seat, scrubbing the mud off the bottoms of his boots before planting them on the skid and the step. Again a wave of nausea grabbed him, but it passed quickly and he felt surprisingly relaxed and steady. This time he knew better what to expect. The animal was almost stationary as he crested the stream bank, and the net enveloped him perfectly like a circus tent.

"That's two!" Buddy sang out.

"That's one," Marc corrected. "Two shots, but one caribou—results, not attempts!"

Greg set down the machine a good distance away from the caribou so they wouldn't traumatize it any more than they had already. The pressure was off. The adrenaline high made Buddy's hands shake so hard he had trouble unhooking the safety harness. Already Marc and Donald were running crouched towards the animal. In their hands, they each carried two fishing tackle boxes containing the collaring and sampling equipment.

Marc eased cautiously behind the entangled bull. Then, with one swift snatch, he grabbed the caribou at the base of its antlers. The animal lunged, but Marc threw his weight against its neck, levering the bull's head down again. Buddy was impressed by the farm-boy technique. Marc was just handling an unruly Four-H Club steer—not rough or violent, simply meeting force with force until eventually the caribou gave up.

Buddy worked the blindfold through the netting, pulled it

over the caribou's eyes and tied the ends off. Unable to see, the bull became momentarily passive, but they knew it could still lash out with hooves honed razor-sharp by winter ice. As a precaution, Donald and Marc slipped a cotton rope around the front feet, then, catching the rear legs with a loop, they drew them tight together.

"Bit like changing a hospital bed—with the patient still in it!" Greg grunted as he used his bear strength, rolling and pulling the large bull, to untangle it from the two nets. Suddenly, with renewed energy, the caribou struggled to break free.

"Hey, knock it off!" Buddy blurted.

"Knock it off?" Marc began laughing. "What the hell? You think you're talking to a trained dog? Man, this is a wild animal! Easy, Abdul!" Marc teased. "Sit, Abdul! Speak, Abdul, speak!"

"Abdul?"

"Goes well with the headdress, don't you think?" Marc pointed to the turban of netting.

Donald slipped the collar around the bull, adjusting it snugly enough that it wouldn't snag on a tree limb, yet loose enough for natural neck expansion during rutting season. The antenna was taped upwards and the transmitter activated by removing a small magnet on the radio housing. Donald turned on his receiver to make sure the collar was sending on the right frequency. Next, Donald began quantifying the animal: measuring the length of the forelegs and diameter of the abdomen. Then he collected samples of feces, hair and even a tooth for determining the animal's age. Finally they untied his feet and Buddy started to undo the blindfold.

"Wait!" Marc exclaimed. "You can't let him go looking like that!" Two long strands of antler velvet draped like sideburns down either side of the caribou's head. Taking out his pocket-knife, Marc trimmed them off. "How about his bangs? Do you think he'd look chic with them raised a couple inches in a page-boy cut?"

"Come on, pull the damn blindfold and let him go. We've harassed him enough in the name of science."

"Science!" Marc laughed sarcastically, "Science? I've seen wolves do cleaner jobs!"

They pulled off the blindfold, then stepped back quickly, giving the bull room to gain his feet. For a minute he just lay there blinking, his eyes adjusting to the light. Then he was up and, after a quick glance around, he bolted towards the stream. But suddenly he stopped and turned towards them. It was an unmistakable look of bewilderment—a "what in the hell did you do that for" kind of look.

Marc bent down and picked up the pieces of antler velvet and some tufts of winter hair that had come off the caribou in the scuffle. "Not very professional." He shook his head, looking at the debris and then at the others on the team. "Not very professional at all!"

They still had enough daylight left for one more capture. After the problems with Abdul, they went for a younger bull with a smaller rack. Twenty minutes after the initial pursuit, they released the caribou fully collared, measured and recorded—a statistic for someone's computer. It was a good way to end the day, and they felt like a team again.

Sitting on a knoll in the middle of the meadow, passing around a thermos cup of coffee, the team took a break from the helicopter before the long flight to base camp. It seemed to Buddy that he could taste the solitude and smell the wilderness as the long, solstice sun cast great shadows off the Aztec-red peaks. Dew collected, releasing the biting aroma of willow, drawing small bands of caribou onto the meadow to feed on the damp marsh grass. It was hard to believe that, just a half hour before, the monastic meadow had resonated with the unholy thunder of technological man unleashed.

"Did you see that parting look Abdul gave us?" Donald laughed.

"He probably couldn't figure us out. After us going to so much work to catch him, and then not eating him!"

"Strange creatures, we humans!" Marc agreed.

"I'll be—there he is!" exclaimed Donald.

"Who?"

"Abdul!" Donald was looking through his binoculars in the

opposite direction from where they had last left the bull. Everyone took turns with the glasses, confirming the radio collar and scrubbed antlers.

"Check out his bangs!" Marc exclaimed. "I told you we should have raised them!"

"Pretty amazing." Greg nodded. "It wasn't so long ago that he was bound and gagged like a common criminal. Now look at him, wild and free as the wind."

"Except that he's bugged," Donald mused. "A spy in the wilderness."

At last the sounds of day gave way to the whispers of night, and the once-muffled murmur of the meadow stream surged into the vacuum. For a long time, no one spoke.

"Yes, yes," Marc said at last with a deep sigh, "we're *very* privileged folks! Very privileged, indeed! " He turned to Buddy. "What's it like hanging out there with the net gun?"

"Religious ecstasy," he wanted to say, but he doubted that the others would understand. They had to be there on the lip of the seat to know. "Terrifying," he said. "Probably about like what a newborn feels, being yarded from the safety of the womb and swung upside down by its heels!" Buddy laughed.

Again they listened to the evening, each absorbed in his thoughts.

"Very privileged, indeed!" Marc sighed, turning to Donald. "But when you write your capture report"—he flashed that grin—"claim that the caribou really love being captured—and we really hate it!"

WITHOUT A TRACE

IT WAS JANET'S MORNING TO SLEEP IN, AND BUDDY WAS MAKING breakfast for the kids when the news came over the radio. No names were given, not even a description of the missing plane, but somehow he knew immediately it was Marc's. Buddy called Donald. He'd had the same premonition.

The provincial search and rescue team arrived in a Buffalo aircraft, and soon Marc's hangar looked like a military command post. Topographical maps were pinned to the walls and divided into sectors with a felt-tip pen. Beside them hung a list of available pilots and spotters and their assigned areas. As Buddy watched the objective, dispassionate professionalism of the rescue co-ordinators, he felt confident that Marc would be found soon, as though the maps somehow made the immense task more possible by qualifying the landscape, making the wild, rugged terrain more approachable.

Search and rescue had become commonplace lately as more and more planes came into the North while weather information remained limited to visuals and radio word of mouth. But the search for Marc was different from the norm. More than a hundred spotters crowded into the hangar that morning, and the airport's aprons became clogged with private planes. Everyone knew Marc. He was their umbilical cord: supplies to the stranded, medicine to the sick, news and messages to the lonely and isolated scattered across the thousands of square miles of northwestern Canadian wilderness.

Box lunches were handed out while the co-ordinating officer, a captain in a blue jump suit with an eagle insignia on the shoulder, briefed them on what to expect. "The first few days will be the most critical. With winter so close, survival chances drop proportionally over time." Buddy could tell that Marc was an object to the man, a lost watch to be found. Still, he was glad someone had a balanced perspective. "Watch for anything out of the ordinary, like a peculiar colour of light off a lake's surface. If a plane goes into water, there are usually oil slicks or fuel leaks of some kind. Also, keep your eyes open for broken treetops and limbs. Often peeled bark will stand out a bright yellow against the green canopy. Smoke is the most obvious sign, either white or black. Sometimes clouds will hang in the timber and look like smoke, but don't assume, always check it out. And don't get into the habit of looking just below you—scan the horizon periodically. But most of all"—his eyes studied the group of spotters—"don't just look where you *want* them to be. Every situation has to be considered!"

As Greg, Donald and Buddy flew the chopper towards their assigned sector, they talked about everything except what was foremost on their minds. Eventually, however, even small talk became so laborious that the conversation died from its own weight.

"Ah, we'll find Marc sitting on some gravel bar, drinking tea and wondering what's taking us so long," Greg concluded as they retreated into their private thoughts.

Buddy remembered the first time he met Marc. Donald had brought Marc into the caribou project for the fixed-wing reconnaissance after a few dozen animals had been collared. Marc's reputation had preceded him—he was by everyone's measure the best bush pilot around.

"Well, folks," Marc had announced as he barged through the cook-house door at base camp (he and Donald had just landed after the first tracking flight), "the wolves won't go hungry this winter!"

Of the thirty-six animals collared, four were dead. All old bulls. It was Donald's guess that the capture drug had left them lethargic, and since wolves are omnipresent opportunists of even slight changes, the tranquillizer had likely tipped the scales in the predators' favour.

"Pretty expensive meat, don't you think?" Marc asked rhetorically as he shook Buddy's hand, not bothering with introductions. "Wouldn't it be a lot cheaper to just fly them in some prime beef cattle?"

If anyone could survive in the bush, Marc could. He was a good pilot. He had the savvy and instincts of a seasoned trapper. But what if he was unconscious? What if.... No, Buddy couldn't allow himself to play the what if game. Someone would find him, just as Greg said, sitting on a sandbar sipping tea. It would be appropriate if *they* found him, after all the team had shared. Still, if the plane had suffered a hard crash, Buddy prayed they wouldn't be the ones to find it.

Most of all, Buddy prayed Marc was alive. He felt hypocritical, for he hadn't prayed since he was a kid when he'd bartered going to church in exchange for God's help catching a particularly big, smart trout. However, when Buddy caught the trout and somehow forgot to go to church, and then went on to catch more trout, he soon lost interest in the exercise. Still, no atheists in foxholes, he affirmed, and again bartered openly.

The hours stretched as the crew strained to see with superhuman vision through the canopy of treetops to the forest floor hundreds of feet below. Rock ledges glared at them, bleak and barren. Steep-sided canyons plunged violently below the helicopter with such abruptness that Buddy winced with the thought of Marc going down there. At least along the rivers or on the bald alpine slopes there was a chance. Down there, there was no hope! A piece of tin flashing on an abandoned trapper's cabin momentarily sparked their hopes. A little later someone spotted a man waving his arms—but it proved to be a boar grizzly standing fiercely on his hind legs, swatting the air as the helicopter passed over his grassy knoll. Mostly it was just hard, raw terrain.

"My eyes are starting to melt," Greg said at last. "Let's set down for lunch on that sandbar."

Each of them took his lunch away from the helicopter to a separate part of the gravel island; each sat looking in a different direction. Buddy stared across the river to the wall of heavy black spruce entangled in a maddening web of devil's club. Marc could be just yards away and they'd never know it. Suddenly something made Buddy shudder. The bush somehow felt dark and foreboding, somehow voracious and evil. He knew better than that. Nature is neutral, he'd learned from experience and Slim and Casey. It was neither good nor bad, kind nor ruthless. There were only events without value except as they pertained to survival. Still, he couldn't shake the feeling of malevolence radiating from the thick jungle across the river. Throwing the rest of his sandwich in the river, Buddy sprang to his feet. Greg was already untying the helicopter's blades.

They followed the river downstream to where it met an ocean fiord south of Bella Bella. Flying north along the sea cliffs, they entered the coastal mountains at the mouth of another of the ubiquitous watersheds and followed it upstream As they searched every side canyon, Buddy realized how the landscape of tall Sitka spruce and polished granite crags could easily absorb a plane without a trace. Hours passed; again Buddy's eyes grew tired.

"There they are!" Buddy shouted as he spotted the white abdomen of the fuselage nestled at the foot of a cliff face in a dwarfed fir stand. Everyone's hopes raced.

"Watch for survivors," Greg said clinically and banked the helicopter hard in anticipation. "If it's Marc, we'll land above him on that open ridge and walk down." But it wasn't him, only the bleached skeleton of a great spruce snag that had fallen over.

In the last light, Greg finally turned the machine towards home. Fuel was getting low, and besides, somebody else had probably found them. The thought was a welcome reprieve from the morose mood that had possessed them throughout the afternoon. Back at base, they went immediately to the hangar. But when the search co-ordinator asked if they'd seen anything, their spirits fell. Dutifully the co-ordinator transferred their flight course onto the map. The Buffalo was still out. Everyone waited. Just at dark the giant craft bellowed onto the tarmac. Nothing.

"Get a good night's sleep and be back here tomorrow, seven o'clock."

"Did you find your friend?" Buddy's oldest daughter asked as he tucked her into bed.

"Tomorrow we'll find him. Tomorrow, for sure," he said convincingly.

Marc had the touch. He knew the bush, and the North was full of stories about bush pilots surviving for weeks, sometimes months under savage conditions. Then one day they'd simply walk out to a road or a trapper's cabin. Not always with all their fingers and toes, but alive!

Looking at his daughter, Buddy remembered a conversation he'd once had with Marc. "It's strange," Marc had said, "how children give us the excuse to be kids again, yet force us to be more adult than we ever thought possible." Suddenly Buddy realized that, above all other things, he wanted to be with his children as they grew up. Then, like a stab from a sharp knife, the idea took a deeper twist as he thought about Marc's two young sons.

"Tomorrow," Buddy repeated himself, "tomorrow we'll find him."

But they didn't find him the next day. Buddy found himself kissing his children good-bye in the morning and hugging them thankfully each evening, with far more emotion than a day's absence warranted. And then there was the recurring dream. They'd flown over Marc's plane, and though he'd built a signal fire, they still hadn't seen him. Buddy would wake with Marc's yells fresh in his head.

Finally, the sector map became covered with flight patterns until there was nowhere that hadn't been covered at least twice. During the search, the wreckage of a plane missing for ten years was found—the bodies had long since been strung across the land by wolves and bears. But not a trace of Marc.

Buddy felt confused standing beside Janet in the doorway to the hangar. It wasn't at all what he'd expected, of course. It had been nine months of long, hollow winter since the search and rescue operation had occupied Marc's hangar. Now the large room was clean and alive, looking more like a country club dining room than a bush plane garage. On the workbench in the back, where once the vital organs of a Beech engine had been strewn, there were dozens of casserole dishes, salads and loaves of bread. A bar was set up in the meat locker, the coldest corner in the building, where previously a blood-matted grizzly hide and a caribou cape had lain waiting to be shipped to a taxidermist. There were spring flower settings, yellow daffodils and white daisies, arranged on the long banquet tables. Ladies in bright dresses and men in jackets, pressed slacks and polished boots visited casually—stark contrasts to the solemn congregation of spotters waiting with tired, raw eyes for the next day's assignments. It's the way Marc would have wanted it, Buddy thought.

There was a wide cross section of northerners present. Indians from Telegraph Creek and outfitters from Yukon. Along the sidelines stood a veritable garden of wallflowers, wilted trappers and weathered prospectors, solemn and alone, watching the gathering like anxious animals. Off to one corner, a tight cluster of hard-rock miners spoke covertly with mine executives about promising core samples and the possibility of stocks soaring on the exchange if word got out.

For many, Marc had been their sole contact with the outside, bringing a human mirror to reflect their sanity—or lack of it, depending on how long they'd been in the bush. Sometimes just buzzing their cabins was enough, checking to see that they were still alive. Someone cared. There would be many stories circulating the hangar that night about how Marc had made a tight landing on a postage-stamp meadow to retrieve a wounded hunter or set down on a snow field to bring mail to a couple isolated for the winter in a mining camp.

And then there were the widows, bush widows and bush-pilot widows, like Henry Willard's wife. It would be five years in August since Henry crashed. As Buddy watched her, he realized something was different, her face had changed. The worry lines that once ran like well-used forest trails while Henry was alive and flying, seemed softer, less travelled. Beside her, Marc's wife, Cheryl, brushed unsuccessfully at her older son's haystack of unruly hair. A younger boy hung on her skirts. Buddy recognized in her eyes the hyperbolic route of anticipation and sadness—that repetitive, manic course through loss, then hope, then emptiness again as the last search plane landed each evening. But then, with the morning flights, the eyes would be rekindled again and begin afresh the downward spiral, until finally there was no reason to hope except out of habit.

Maybe he, too, had the look, Buddy thought: he hadn't fully adjusted to the fact that there was no hope. Still, he was glad he'd come. He always liked the hangar. It had been the jumping-off point to many adventures for him. He envisioned the building as a kind of time depot, an intersection between the present and the past, where travellers arrived in jets from Vancouver— from the world made in man's image—and departed in bush planes for Spartan camps in the northern wilderness, where man's presence was tenuous at best, and easily swallowed in the mosaic of mountains and alluvial valleys. Hunters and fishermen would come through the hangar from Europe and the east coast of the States. Dressed in their Abercrombie and Fitch camouflage suits and great down jackets, they looked like khaki versions of the Pillsbury doughboy. How differently they'd return, Buddy had mused, their clothes filthy with pine pitch and animal blood, pungent with the smell of campfire smoke. On their faces a stump farm of stubble grew, and their eyes were perplexed and disoriented; space travellers, Buddy thought, from a world of timeless silence, cast into a world deafened by noise.

"Are those Marc's parents?" Janet asked, pointing towards an older couple standing near the head table. The man was tall and gangly, looking shy and awkward in a black suit that Buddy suspected hadn't been off its hanger in years. The woman, short and heavy set, wore a pale print dress and a pink cotton jacket. Both were in their mid-sixties and both had the same tempered Slavic features and prairie farmer complexions—a wheat farm north of Regina, to be exact.

Beside the couple stood a striking woman in a suede dress. Susanne, Marc's sister, had inherited the stature and cheekbones of her father and the gentle eyes and soft mouth of her mother. But there was something about Susanne that Buddy found disturbing, a strange melancholy. She was talking to Dereck, her younger brother.

"Welcome, strangers!" Dereck greeted Buddy and Janet. Buddy was startled to realized how much Dereck had grown to look like Marc. "I'm glad you could come. Mom and Dad were asking about you. Susanne's here. She and her husband flew up from the States. Oh, did you see the plaque, Buddy?" He pointed to a large piece of polished marble set in front of the head table. "We're going to mount it at the end of the airstrip at your base camp up north. We think it's more appropriate up there in the mountains than down here in a cemetery. Don't you?"

Janet detached herself to visit with Marc's parents. Buddy got a drink and returned to the plaque. The marble headstone had an embossed metal picture of Marc on it, and of course he was grinning that goddamn grin. Buddy smiled and lifted his glass. "To you, Cloud Walker." It was a nickname they'd given him for his passion of prowling the sky. Marc had two ways to fly, depending upon his clients. For most passengers, it was bus service—climb to altitude, then fly from A to B, door to door. But alone, or with those who asked for it, he flew as if he were riding a horse: checking for wildlife along the valley bottoms, slipping up a ridge to see what was roaming around the rim rock. Reading tracks from the air as though they were written on flight maps. Not dangerous flying, but close enough to know the land intimately, giving it face and history.

Standing there in front of the plaque, Buddy recalled their last flight together. It was fall, a few weeks before Marc went missing. They'd finished a big collaring program with just enough time to get out of base camp before winter storms began rolling in from the coast. The sky was clear when they lifted off from the airstrip, but as Marc's Cessna flew out of the valley they discovered a storm front building to the west. Soon the shrouds of hag's hair clouds swept in around them. Greg was still at base camp with the helicopter, but he warned them over the radio not to return, that the visibility had deteriorated to zero. No place to go but forward. Marc shrugged. He circled the plane at the entrance to a mountain pass that led into another watershed. Spreading a topographic map across his lap, he looked at his watch.

"We'll follow this creek"—he pointed to the map—"to the divide. And there we'll pick up the Skeena headwaters and take it out the other side." Then he grinned that grin. "Keep your eyes open through the pass, we might get lucky and spot some animals."

Buddy laughed, though there was little humour in it. The driving snow made it impossible to see anything straight ahead. What little visibility they had was directly below. Buddy knew it was going to be blind-faith flying, listening to the drone of the engine, wondering if it was propelling them safely through the divide—or head-on against an unseen mountain.

"Marshmallow clouds with granite centres." Marc sang a Mark Perry song.

The minutes passed agonizingly slowly for Buddy as they flew above the diminishing cord of water, until finally it was just a faint thread. Buddy's nerves were frayed; his heart raced because he knew from the topographics that the rock walls of the adjacent mountains must be right beside them. When he felt like he'd explode from the tension, even the thin string of running water stopped in a high alpine swamp separating watersheds.

Then a fresh line of water appeared and began swelling and finally cascading joyously out of the basin. "Once again we've thwarted death!" Marc smiled, never really believing otherwise.

"Do you remember that rhubarb cobbler Marc made at base camp?" Greg said as he and Donald came up beside Buddy in front of the plaque.

"God, it was awful! What did he do, forget the sugar or something?"

"No sugar, " Donald snorted. "And to make matters worse, he used straight flour and water for the cake. It reminded me of lumps of moose shit floating on an algae swamp!"

"You know, I think it's still sitting on the windowsill at base camp. He left it there last fall to soak—should be good and tender by now!" It felt good to laugh again.

"God, it seems like a lifetime ago."

The speeches and tributes for Marc began after dinner, with dessert and coffee. But Buddy felt uneasy. He didn't want things capsulated so fast, wrapped up in a tight package, leaving behind only the memory of memories—not yet, anyway. He slipped outside for a cigarette.

It was a black, obsidian night, hard and impenetrable and revealing more of oneself than the night. Buddy sat down on an ore crate beside the hangar. In the distance he thought he heard the drone of a plane but he wasn't sure. It would be strange if it were, since the runway lights had been turned off for an hour. Possibly it was a trick played by the mind upon a susceptible imagination. Buddy knew how desire could whisper sounds in one's ears. As a boy, wrangling horses in the early morning, he'd strain to hear their bells until soon they'd be ringing clear and loud in his ears—even though there wasn't an animal for miles. Now, as then, he stretched his senses.

"Oh, here you are." Janet stepped out the hangar door, the heat and sounds of the party inside enveloping her. "The band's setting up."

"I'll be in soon, I was just having a cigarette."

Janet sat down beside him, for a long time saying nothing.

"Buddy, I don't know if you'll hear this, but it's got to be said and tonight's as good a time as any." She hesitated as though drawing her courage, then suddenly she turned on him. "I'm sick and tired of your grief!" Her voice snapped with anger. "For nine months I've indulged it and now I'm sick of it! You've become a cancer on our family, always sullen and moody. Even the children know something's wrong with you, and they think it's their fault! In fact, sometimes you act like you blame me!" Again she paused. "Damn it, if you're going to stop living, and wallow in self-pity, do it away from us!"

"What the fuck do you know about it!" Buddy snapped. "What do you know about putting your life in somebody's hands, sharing the same risks day after fucking day, and then they just disappear like they never existed? Let me tell you—"

"No!" Janet cut him off. "Let me tell you! You're not mourning Marc any more; you stopped grieving for him a long time ago. The truth is, you're mourning yourself and your own mortality! Suddenly you see you're going to die, and it scares you!" Her eyes flashed in the lights of the hangar. "You guys were a bunch of high-tech cowboys, riding an edge thinner than any of you knew or cared to look at, all the time believing that because you got to play around in the sky, you were invincible, immortal, like some kind of gods. But then, when you find out you're human just like the rest of us"—Janet jammed a finger against his chest—"you can't handle it! No, you're not grieving for Marc, you're crying for yourself. And I'm sick and tired of it!"

Buddy wanted to strike back in defence, but he caught himself. He knew she was right. Janet had simply given words to the thoughts he'd avoided. In the ensuing silence Buddy understood that she was pleading for him to finally acknowledge the truth. But his ideas rushed around like startled chickens beneath a hawk's shadow, and he couldn't.

"Go to hell!" she finally blurted. "Give me the keys to the truck, I'm going home. You can stay here and freeze, for all I care."

Buddy jerked the keys from his leather jacket and threw them at her.

"That's real mature of you!" she said and slammed the door behind her.

The tables had been moved, and couples danced to the gentle saxophone wail of the Hi-Tones.

"Dance with me, Buddy," said a linear blonde, an old girl friend of Marc's. Though now happily married, she'd gladly give up everything if Marc would walk through the door. Or so she said, but she'd been drinking.

"He was so full of life." Her pretty face brightened. "Never cold and raw like most men who live with the North inside them. He was like a warm coastal breeze sweeping over me from someplace tropical, so easygoing and full of fragrances.

He was always excited about what he was doing, where he was going." Her thoughts left her words behind. "Forgive me," she apologized, "I'm a little drunk."

"You're also a lot sober," Buddy said comfortingly, "but don't worry about it, tonight is the night to let loose our feelings."

"Funny," she continued after a few minutes of slow dancing with her thoughts, "one night in bed, he sat bolt upright from a nightmare. And you know, Buddy, he was really spooked! I think he somehow saw how it was going to end for him—like maybe he saw his own death." Her fingernails sank into Buddy's shoulder, then abruptly she released her grip and walked away.

Buddy joined Marc's sister, Susanne, at the bar. He found it interesting that, during the evening, she'd gravitated towards the "bush" side of Marc's friends, purposefully separating herself from her husband, an American whose passions seemed to be golf and indulging his wife.

"That's a beautiful dress," Buddy said. "I doubt that it's off a rack from the Hudson's Bay Company, is it?"

"Neiman-Marcus," she answered, seemingly out of habit, but quickly smiled, a little embarrassed by her response. "Funny, as a kid, I dreamt about a charge account at a big exclusive store like Neiman-Marcus. That was all I ever wanted in the whole world, or so I thought back then. And now"—she tasted her drink, then looked at it as if it were evidence of her words—"it's all come true!" Again Buddy thought he glimpsed the look of melancholy.

"Lately I get to wondering"—she was talking as much to herself as to him—"if there shouldn't be more?"

"Like what?"

"Risks," she said with no explanation. She changed the subject. "I guess you knew Marc about as well as anyone."

"Everyone knew Marc well." Buddy laughed. "To know him at all was to know him well."

"Marc always had a lot of friends. Even back when we were kids, he was the most popular guy in school. He always acknowledged people and encouraged them to be just what they wanted to be. Once, back on the farm one summer, the three of us kids were all sitting around on the porch, bored to distraction while Mom and Dad were off in the field threshing. I was only seven or eight at the time, which would make Marc about ten, and Dereck couldn't have been more than five or six. Anyway, Dereck was watching this big sow we had, and he asked why people didn't ride pigs like they do horses. Then I wondered out loud what it would be like to ride a pig. And bang, the scales tip. 'Let's do it!' Marc cried—so we did.

"God, I laughed till I peed my pants." The shadow lifted from Susanne's face. "But it didn't matter much. We were so dirty when that pig got through with us, Mom said she'd have to peel off our skin to get us clean." Again she laughed. "Course we weren't really scared, but we still high-tailed it to the river and jumped in, clothes and all."

Buddy tried to imagine what Susanne looked like back then, but the distance between the little farm girl and the stately woman was too great.

"Would you like to dance?" Buddy asked.

"Not really." She smiled. "But I wouldn't mind taking a walk."

As they walked down the darkened runway, Susanne remembered the afternoon Marc took his first plane ride. "Being raised on a farm in the middle of nowhere, we'd never seen a plane up close until I was maybe twelve. It was the year the farm agent talked Dad into hiring a crop duster to fertilize. Maybe that's where Marc went wrong," she said, still caught in the happiness of her memories. "Maybe if his first flight had been a boring, commercial red-eye special with a bitchy stewardess, who knows? He might still be driving a tractor in Saskatchewan. But not Marc. No, sir. He pleaded, flattered, even threatened the pilot until he got a ride in that plane. And as I remember it, the guy was this ragged-edged alcoholic who only marginally gave a squat if he was upside down or right side up anyway." She laughed. "Which suited Marc just fine.

"They came over the house so close we thought they'd hit the top of a big cottonwood there in the front yard. Mom was just beside herself for worrying. She swore she'd put a stop to that nonsense once and for all as soon as they landed. Course, when she saw Marc come running up the road yelling about what he'd seen and done, I guess she knew it was a lost cause." Susanne paused for a long time. "You know, even if Marc had known he'd die in a plane, I doubt he'd have changed."

They walked for a while. "The problem is, a person with so much life in him doesn't die in isolation!" Susanne stopped abruptly. "We all die a little. But you know what the worst part is, Buddy? It's the missing. That's the worst. It's like a sentence without punctuation at the end, just a vague question mark holding his place. It's never knowing how he died or where . . . or even if he's dead. Hell!" Her voice was sharp and angry. "If I only knew for sure that he *is* dead! Oh, I know that sounds crazy—of course he's dead, nine months of fierce northern winter. But somewhere way down inside me where I guess the light of reason doesn't shine, I *still* sometimes feel he's alive."

Buddy knew the feeling. Countless times he'd been working outside and heard the whine of a twin engine. Involuntarily he'd look up, thinking, "It's Marc!" Somehow Marc had patched the plane together and finally come home. That was more consistent with the man than simply going missing.

"Do you get out in the bush much?" Susanne asked.

"Not much."

She stopped, astonished. "Why?"

Buddy felt uncomfortable. "You know how it is, the family and the ranch. I'm hoping to write more. . . ." But he trailed off, aware that his reasons were masks. "The truth is, I'm afraid!" Buddy suddenly blurted, startled to hear himself finally saying it. "The bush is evil!" He sensed that she didn't understand. How could she? He didn't really understand.

"All my life," Buddy said, thinking as he spoke, "nothing charged my batteries like the bush. It was my fuel, my solace, who knows, maybe even my god. Watching an avalanche snap trees like twigs, or listening to a thunderstorm marching through the mountains, echoing off the cliffs like cannons. Somehow all that blind power made me relish my own insignificance." He paused, wondering if she understood. "The wilderness gave me courage, inspiration. To me, watching a monkshood, driven by some unconscious molecular force, push itself up through the first cracks in the spring ice, was a metaphor for the force of the universe itself. But now.... Now I feel...." Buddy hesitated again, searching for a way to say it right. "I feel betrayed!"

"Betrayed?" Susanne asked, confused. "Betrayed by what? By the bush, by God? That's a little presumptuous, isn't it?" Then she checked herself.

"I know. And you're right."

"Buddy," she said after they'd walked for some time in silence, "the wilderness was Marc's freedom. It was his escape from a world of man's making. But he also understood, probably better than anyone else, that the bush is unforgiving. Marc was the one who flew out the bodies. He knew the tremendous toll claimed by the North. But that sure didn't hold him back." Her voice trailed off. "Maybe—and I hope this doesn't sound patronizing—but maybe you've conjured up a safety net that was never there."

"That's the second time tonight someone's told me that." Buddy smiled.

Susanne stopped walking. She turned and took both his hands, their fingers interlocked with the grip of two climbers crossing a crevasse. "Besides, if nature is, as you say, your solace, then you don't really have much choice, do you? I think you just have to accept that it makes you both immortal *and* mortal, and go on with your dreams."

"You sound like your brother."

Susanne sighed; her grip tightened. "Buddy, he *is* dead, isn't he?" she whispered. "And we're never going to know how." For a long time they stood there, sharing their loss. "But tonight we have to bury him!"

Buddy gazed up at the night sky. Once they were away from the glare of the hangar lights, it was so clear they could see stars from horizon to horizon.

"Look there!" Buddy pointed to the north and the vivid green and yellow curtains of aurora borealis rolling and spiking across the sky.

Susanne looked up at the northern lights. "God, it's so quiet and peaceful."

Buddy listened, then realized he no longer heard the drone of the plane.

IN SEARCH OF A SADDLE

"*BUENOS DÍAS, SEÑORES,*" THE MEXICAN ADUANA OFFICER GREETED Buddy and Slim as Slim's ancient Ford Bronco slumped to a derelict stop and gave an emphysemic cough in front of the adobe border station. "*Para dónde va?*"

"Punto Lindo," Buddy replied.

"*Sí?*" The guard looked suspiciously at the two men. It was obvious they were neither engineers nor workers at the Punto Lindo power station. Buddy's hair was long and pulled back in a braid. Slim, wearing a well-travelled cowboy hat and dressed in a shirt and pants that hung on his skeletal frame like a parachute, was obviously too old. "*Porqué Punto Lindo?*" the Mexican asked suspiciously.

"We're gonna get a saddle." Slim leaned across the seat to speak to the man through Buddy's window. Buddy had a sinking feeling in his stomach. If Slim got off on the story, they'd be there the rest of the day.

"*Bueno.*" The guard smiled, accepting the five-dollar bill Buddy pressed into his hand. "Mexico makes many saddles." He puffed out his chest. "Best in the world, *señor. Buena suerte.*" And he waved them through.

"You shouldn't have bribed him," Slim said gruffly to Buddy. "We ain't got nothing to hide."

"Hmm." Buddy grinned. "Except maybe this rig of yours." He tapped the steering wheel of the Bronco. "It's about as legal as a three-dollar bill! Besides," Buddy said with a snort, "what would we say, we're looking for a saddle you lost seventy years ago?"

"I didn't lose it," Slim corrected him. "I just left it. There's a big difference—I know where it is."

"I hope so, Grandpa." Buddy looked earnestly at his grandfather. "But you've got to remember, things have changed a lot in the last seventy years."

"Humph." Slim snorted. "Ain't a day goes by that I don't see that for sure, son. But mountains don't change so much, unless they've been bulldozed down. We'll find that saddle," he added confidently.

Lost or left, it didn't matter. The last thing Buddy wanted was a Mexican Aduana agent rummaging through the trash that cluttered Slim's old Ford. Since Ethel died twelve years ago, Slim had adopted the housekeeping habits of a pack rat. Buddy knew for certain that somewhere rolling around on the floor was a Prince Albert tobacco tin with a couple of dozen dynamite caps clattering loose like a very dangerous marimba rattle. And he was just as sure that somewhere there would be an equal number of forty-per-cent dynamite sticks, either fallen down in the wheel well or wedged under the back seat or covered with so much dust and debris that they lay unnoticed directly underfoot. Caps and dynamite. Buddy laughed. Slim and Casey considered them essential day-to-day tools, like a wrench or a hammer. They used dynamite sometimes instead of an axe, and always instead of a shovel. Buddy remembered spending a lot of time as a kid scratching around for dirt to backfill fence post holes dug with explosives.

Oh, well, Buddy thought as he drove down the hot, liquid asphalt highway flowing south, they were in Mexico now. Going across the border into the United States with the explosives might be another matter, but he'd worry about that when the time came.

Half an hour south of the border, Buddy turned off the pavement and onto a gravel road running northwest, back towards the Rio Grande and Texas. A thick cloud of dust billowed behind them, choking the radiant midday sun in their wake. Before them, the desert shimmered with heat snakes, dissolving the horizon into a mirage of interconnected lakes with cactus islands leaping from their grease-slick surfaces. It was spring, and the desert, mummified by the heat for eleven arid months of the year, suddenly pulsed with thunderstorms, flash floods, and life. Even the wizened, bone-dead cacti rejoiced with flowers and fruit.

"Seems odd being here again after all these years." Slim looked out the open window at the once familiar landscape. "I remember days it got so hot that we'd have to squat in the shade of our horses for shelter. Sometimes, riding day herd, you'd think the air was gonna hit its flash point, and the whole desert would ignite like the head of a match."

"Grandpa," said Buddy, "tell me the saddle story again."

"The saddle story," Slim repeated, thinking for a moment. "Well, let's see." He leaned against the seat, the back of his Stetson curling up as it pressed against the rear window. "It was around nineteen-aught-four, I believe. I was working just north of here for the King ranch, there across the border in Texas. My job was riding range and doctoring a herd of cows for ticks and for cuts they'd get from the mesquite brush. But this one time, the King brothers sent me and a partner of mine named Clovus down across the border into Old Mexico to buy back a running-brand herd."

"What's a running-brand herd?" Buddy interrupted.

"One that's been rustled." Slim smiled. "But we wasn't the rustlers. We was just buying back cattle from this Mexican who'd acquired them with some artistic branding on a cloudy night. But back then, the King boys didn't give much never mind, even if they was sometimes buying back their own cows. They just wanted livestock for the homestead land they was swindling away from the government with counterfeit settlers. In fact"—the old man laughed—"somewhere there in Texas, there's a quarter section with my name on the original title."

"Maybe it's got oil on it and you're filthy rich," Buddy teased.

"Wouldn't do me no good. I sold it to the King boys for a silver dollar—that was the agreement. Anyway, like I was saying, the King boys didn't pay no never mind that the cows was stolen, but the Texas Rangers sure did!"

"How do you mean?"

"Well, as I recall, we was about half a day south of the Rio Grande, coming back with maybe forty scruff cows, when these two Rangers got on our tail. We knowed it was Rangers by the way they turned onto our tracks like wolves following bloody meat. Course, with them cows ahead of us, we weren't making no headway at all, so we decided to cut loose the herd and each of us high-tail it off in a different direction." The old cowboy shook his head. "Well, dern the luck, *both* those Ranger boys come after me.

"They had pretty fair ponies, I must say. And mine was just a drag-ass cow pony, and I figured for sure I was about to be a guest of the state. But then I spied a train far off to the south climbing real slow up this long hill. It gave me an idea, and I lit out after it at a full gallop. I could see where this arroyo swung close to the tracks, so I turned my horse down into it and galloped along the bottom of the ravine till I figured I was near the rail grade. Then I stripped the saddle and bridle off my horse and sent him high-tailing on up the arroyo. I pitched the gear into a washout cave back in the bank and hid myself in some mesquite just below the rim of the ravine. And it was there, while I was waiting for the train, that I took a bearing off the west shoulder of the two mesas to give me a line back to where I'd hid the saddle. The Rangers rode right on by like they was supposed to, but pretty soon they figured out what I'd done, and they came back just as I made my run for the train. Oh, they fired off a couple rounds in my general direction, but they didn't mean nothing by 'em. I figure, if they was fixing to hit me, I'd've been dead about then."

As Buddy looked at the desert, he imagined the young cowboy running for the train, swinging onto a boxcar, his chaps flapping like startled sage grouse. Ever since he was a kid, sitting in the evening with his grandfather on the back porch of the lodge in Wyoming, Buddy had heard the Texas stories. They were his bedtime stories. Now they had substance and meaning. Expecting Slim to continue, Buddy glanced over at his grandfather. But the old man's chin rested on his chest, his Stetson bowing and lifting with the rhythm of his snoring.

Buddy was glad he'd come, even though it wasn't a particularly good time to leave British Columbia and the research project. They'd just got a grant to radio collar four grizzly bear and monitor them along with the caribou the team had previously tagged. Spring was the best time to capture grizzly, when they were exposed up on the alpine stalking caribou calves and marmots. Still, when his grandfather asked him along, Buddy knew he couldn't refuse. This might well be their last trip together—Slim was eighty-four that January. And even though the old man's brain was purring right along, Buddy could tell that his body, like his Bronco, was worn out.

Also, though Slim would never admit it, he *needed* Buddy. For one thing, Buddy knew that Slim needed him to drive. Slim thought he drove perfectly well with just one eye. The retina had been torn on the other eye by a colt Slim was breaking. But the motor vehicle bureau didn't feel the same way. And two years ago, they'd refused to renew the old man's driver's licence. It was about the same time the Bronco failed its safety inspection, so its licence plates were expired—as was its insurance. Blind, illegal and uninsured, yet somehow Slim got away with it, at least in Skyline, where the rules were bent out of respect for the old man. But driving across the country was a different matter. "What they gonna do to me?" Slim would argue whenever Buddy mentioned the subject. "Throw an old man in jail and run the risk of me dying there? And I'm just contrary enough to do it." But, given Slim's passion for dynamite, Buddy had other concerns. For years Buddy had been expecting a telephone call informing him that Slim had had a highway accident, blowing to bits a few innocent people plus a goodly section of the countryside in the process.

They came to a junction in the gravel road. A large blue and white sign smiled down upon them. *Campesino* children gazed transfixed at a brilliant light bulb with the adoration normally reserved for crucifixes and Madonna shrines. Beneath the picture, the message proclaimed the benefits of the thermal-electrical coal-burning generator at Punto Lindo, down the left fork fourteen miles. Buddy's gaze travelled the road until it disappeared into an adobe-brown haze. The alternative, the road to the right, veered off to the east towards a single mesa rising from the desert floor like a lone stump of a monolithic tree.

"Grandpa." He shook the old man lightly. "Which way?"

Slim came erect in the seat with a start. He blinked, adjusting to the sun off the sand. "I wasn't sleeping. Just resting my eyes. Which way?" he repeated the question. "What does the sign say? I ain't got my glasses," he said, even though he couldn't read Spanish anyway.

"It says they are lighting the way to the future," Buddy said sarcastically. "But judging by that smog, I'd say they're just polluting it. But that isn't why I woke you up. Look over there." He pointed to the east and the mesa. "Is that what you're looking for?"

For a long time, Slim studied the mountain. "I think that's the one closest to the railroad grade. But where's the second one? Don't you recall? There was two of 'em."

"Lost in the haze of the future, I suspect." Buddy nodded towards the power station. He looked at the Bronco's gas gauge. There was still three-quarters of a tank. He turned the rig onto the track running east towards the mesa.

"Grandpa, what made you leave your home there in Mississippi?"

"What, more stories? That last one was so dull it even put *me* to sleep." Slim frowned, though Buddy could tell he was pleased to be asked about the stories.

"Well, I was thirteen when I left home. Some say that's too young to start making it on your own, but I didn't have no choice in the matter, I was running for my life."

"Running for your life?"

"That's exactly right. What happened was, me and an older brother named Whit was plowing with a team of mules on the folks' farm there in Union, Mississippi. Whit was a real mean son of a bitch, mean to us young'ns, mean to the animals, boy-howdy." Slim scowled.

"Anyway, I was at the head leading the team, and Whit was on the plow handles, when the blade come hard against this rock—must'a been the size of a cabin cuz it near jerked the team off their feet. Course, when the plow dug down, the handles jumped up and they flipped Whit ass over teakettle. Flew so high, he landed flat on his back four furrows away... knocked the wind right out of him! Well." Slim grunted. "When he come up, he was plumb crazy, and right off he starts beating the mules around the head with the reins and all, like it was their fault.

"Humph." Slim snorted. "That was all she wrote! I'd tolerated about as much as I could of that man, and I grabbed me a hickory limb about the size of a baseball bat and laid a lick against the side of Whit's head just as hard as I could swing. He dropped like a dead steer. But unfortunately, he *weren't* dead, and I know'd when he come conscious again, he'd kill me if he caught me. So I took that limb again and I give him a smack in the leg for safe measure so he wouldn't chase me. Then I took off with just the clothes on my back. And I ain't never been back."

"So how did you end up in Wyoming?" Buddy asked.

"Well, first I caught a cotton train down to Biloxi, and then a freight to New Orleans. Worked there as a riveter's helper on a bridge over the Mississippi until we reached the other side and the job ended. Then I hitched a ride upriver to Shreveport on a paddle wheeler hauling Caribbean rum north. That was the first time I'd ever tasted alcohol that didn't come from a still." Slim laughed.

"Finally in Shreveport I got a steady job at a livery stable. The family that owned it didn't have no young'ns so they kinda took me in for a year, gave me a little education and all. But somehow I just couldn't picture myself cooped up in Louisiana for the rest of my natural days. So finally I thanked them for all they'd done and hit the trail again. Rode the rails, mainly, till I wound up on the King ranch."

"And I probably would've stayed in Texas if it weren't for a fall in cattle prices, that and poor spring pasture. As it turned out, the King boys figured to move their yearling steers north. But instead of taking the Chisholm Trail to Kansas like normal, they decided to drive the herd up through New Mexico and Colorado to the railhead at Cheyenne, and fatten them up along the way. I was sixteen at the time, and son, let me tell you, that was sure some drive. One hundred and four days in the saddle, sleeping on the ground, eating salt pork and pinto beans—unless of course a steer broke its leg, then we was nursing on the fat tit. But the worst part was the cross fencing. It was a bad deal, and a couple of men even got killed over that damn stuff. One of them I knowed real well," Slim remembered. "Oh, I don't fault the farmers for putting it up, but I sure hope that one day in hell I meet the guy who come up with that idea for barbed wire!"

Slim sat for a long time looking out the side window.

"And?" Buddy asked.

"And," Slim returned to the story, "it was late August when we finally rode into Cheyenne. The railroad was planning a real big haul east with three trains pulling fifty cattle cars each, and there must have been two thousand head of cows total. There was herds and cowhands from as far north as Alberta, and of course we'd come from about as far south as you could come without eating tacos for breakfast. There was a couple guys from Skyline who I got on with pretty good, and the way they talked up the country and all, I considered going up there and having a look for myself. They said there was plenty of work for a man with a saddle. Unfortunately, at the time I didn't have one. I'd been riding a borrowed one from the King boys. And my prospects for getting one with my meagre trail wages was nigh on to none.

"But as it turned out, while we was all there in Cheyenne, sorting out the cattle and the likes, word come around that the Flying W Ranch and the Sweetgrass Cattle Company—they was big cattle brokers at the time—plus the town of Cheyenne was sponsoring a rodeo and barbecue. And to boot, they was offering good money and new saddles for prizes.

"Mind you, in them days rodeo was just two events, roping and bronc busting. And to tell the truth, Buddy, I never was one to throw a rope very fast or straight. So I signed up for the bronc busting.

"Weren't no arena. Just narrow sorting corrals that opened out onto a chunk of God's own property stretching unhindered clear to the horizon. And as I recall, the bucking chute was just a swing gate hinged onto the outside planks of the fence. What they'd do is sandwich a bronc between the corral and the gate just long enough for a cowboy to get on—then it was Katie bar the door! Oh, there was a few buggies and the odd automobile stationed out across the sagebrush in a rough circle. I guess they was supposed to be deterrents for runaways. But in truth, they was more of a hindrance than a help, cuz the poor horses was more scared of cars than they was of the cowboy on their backs."

Slim leaned back against the Ford's seat. "The first horse I drew weren't much, but I stayed with him and the judges moved me up in the competition. My next horse was a dern sight better, and I made good honest points on him, at least good enough to move onto the finals. But, Buddy, that last bronc!" The old man grinned. "Son, I ain't never to this day drawn better. Boy-howdy, he was a horse and a half! I can recall him clear as can be: a big buckskin with a powerful thick chest and a boxed-up ass, and all the fury of a tornado trapped in a horse's hide. When he exploded out of the gate, I swear, he lunged halfway across that field on the first jump! Then, don't you know, he sucked back like the tip of a cracking bullwhip, and if I hadn't had my spurs high on his shoulders from the start, he would've thrown me clear down to Colorado. Wowee." Slim whistled, shaking his head. "But like I said, I caught his rhythm on the first buck and I stayed right with him. And from then on, I was sitting on a porch swing with my sweetheart. And just to show the judges I was glued on tight, I started fanning him with my hat and even stayed with him a few jumps after they blowed the bugle." Slim's eyes sparkled. "It weren't my intention to show off, but the minute I hit the ground, I let out this great big yahoo, cuz I know'd it was about as fine a ride as I was ever going to make in my life." He smiled, and the creases in his face folded into deep canyons. "I guess the judges thought so, too, cuz they give me some pretty high marks."

Buddy had seen his grandfather make some pretty good rides over the years, yet this was the one that stayed in the old man's memory.

"But then, don't you know, just a couple of riders later, another feller draws another showy pony and he rides it right through to the end, too. Well, after I'd seen what a good job he'd done, I just says to myself that there ain't no shame losing to a ride like that, and I began packing my gear. But the judges turned around and gave him exactly the same number of points as me.

"Course, the sponsors come to us and asked if we'd be interested in a ride off, winner take all—fifty dollars cash and a new Form Fitter Hieser saddle. Well, I figured I weren't never going to improve on my last ride, so I told the other fellow that if he had a like mind, I was willing to split the proceeds. Since he had a wife and a passel of young'ns, I said to him, 'Why don't you take the money, you got a *need* for it and all I got is *wants*. But I could sure use that saddle if that seemed a fair swap.' So that's what we done."

"And that's when you went to Skyline?" Buddy asked.

"Pretty much. It seemed like right after the rodeo and the trains pulled out, the town suddenly took a dim view of cowhands hanging around. And the sheriff's office begun arresting cowboys right and left for vagrancy. One day, I recall this deputy stopped me on the street and asked if I got any friends in Cheyenne. And I know'd he didn't mean cowboy friends.

" 'Yes, sir,' I said, 'I got ten of them!' and I reached in my pocket and showed him ten silver dollars, the last of my summer's wages. Well, don't you know, he looked at them and started laughing and just sent me on about my business. But I know'd it was time to move on, so I hooked up with those two cowboys from Skyline, and I guess you know the rest." Slim leaned back, reflecting.

"Sometimes I wonder," he said after a long silence, "just what would've happened if I'd taken that money instead. Maybe it would've gone good for me—maybe not. But you know, Buddy," he said, looking at his grandson, "I just can't imagine any better life than the one me and Ethel had there in Skyline."

Neither man spoke for a long while. Finally Slim reached over and turned on the radio and tried to tune in a station. But all he could find was a Texas station that was wrestling for the same frequency with a local Mexican *cantina*-brass station. Finally, he grew impatient with the noise and abruptly shut the radio off.

"Dern the music you kids listen to nowadays," he grumbled. Buddy didn't try to explain.

"Your daddy was a pretty fair rodeo hand in his own right," Slim reflected as he watched the mesa take on detail the closer they got.

"I heard he was invited to the nationals once," Buddy probed. "But that there was something about Dad and a cousin named Katie. I asked Jep if he knew anything, but he just dodged the question and did his silent-Indian routine. What did happen exactly?"

Slim shifted, his eyes narrowing. "By all rights, son, your daddy should be the one to tell you." He thought for a moment. "But I guess it don't matter much now. He's put them days behind him a long time ago." Buddy suspected Slim was talking about the time Casey was committed to the psychiatric hospital. "Him and your mammy, Sheila, has done a good job running the ranch, don't you think?" the old man asked.

"They must, the guests keep coming back every year."

"You know, don't you, that your daddy and me always figured you'd take over the business when you returned from college," Slim said, but Buddy cut him off.

"Grandpa, we've been over that. It isn't the same any more." He hesitated, but decided not to make an issue of it. "It seems to me that what folks call wilderness now is just glorified parks where you got to take out a permit to piss. That's not for me and Janet. We want what you had, animals that are afraid of man."

"Did you find it in Canada?"

"At first, for a while anyway. Now the clear-cuts and the dams are starting to eat up the wilderness pretty fast. But that's another subject. You were telling me about Dad, remember?"

"To tell you the truth, I don't to this day understand it all," Slim confessed. "One summer, Casey worked the rodeo circuit real hard so he could qualify for the nationals. But then when he got an invite to the competition, he just didn't show up for either of his horses. First thing we heard for sure was a call from our niece, Katie Haynes. She said Casey was staying with her there in Denver." Slim frowned. "Well, that sat hard with Ethel and me, since we knowed Katie was whoring herself out at the time. Also, Ethel figured Katie was drunk when she called. Then, when your grandmammy asked to talk with Casey, I gather he went kinda funny in the head, and I guess that's when the police put him in the hospital.

"Naturally, I dropped everything I was doing and went down there in the De Soto. But Buddy"—Slim's tone suddenly softened—"when I seen him there in the hospital, I got to tell you, I just had to cry. He was sure in sorry shape. Looked like a beaten dog, all curled up in a corner of this little room with bars over the window. He didn't recognize me at all, didn't even seem to see me. It was like someone had thrown a switch in his brain." There was a note of sadness in Slim's voice. "It was a long, long time before he started coming around. And in the end, when the doctors gave up, it was Ethel who finally got him out of there. Then your mammy come along, and your daddy's been fine ever since."

"What happened to Katie Haynes?"

"Now there's a strange story. A few months after they'd committed Casey, Ethel and me gets a letter from her on real nice stationery. She says she's gonna get married to a rancher in Green River Station around the middle of November, and could we drive over for the wedding.

"We didn't bear her no grudge. Fact, we was real happy for her; she'd had a pretty tough row to hoe in life. But we just couldn't get away from the ranch at the time, so Ethel wrote back to the Denver address apologizing, and she included a white lace veil Katie's mammy had made for Ethel when we got hitched years ago. Don't know if Katie ever got it.

"Anyway, the next thing we know is when word come to us around the end of November that she was dead, froze to death on her wedding night, if you can imagine. They said she and her husband was headed out in a blizzard to his sheep ranch after the wedding, and they skidded off the road. According to the story, he went for help, but by the time he got back a couple hours later, she was dead."

"That's strange." Buddy frowned. "People don't generally die that fast if they've got shelter."

"Course not, and that's what's crazy about the affair. They say she froze cuz the windshield was blown out—by a shotgun blast—from the inside!"

Buddy stared at Slim, astonished.

"At first they arrested her husband cuz it was his gun, but that didn't make no sense. Killing your wife on your wedding night? As it finally turned out, the sheriff's office ruled it was accidental, figuring she must've accidentally shot off the gun herself. But I guess only God will ever know what went through that poor girl's mind." He gazed out the window. "To my way of thinking, Katie died from the same disease that takes a lot of prairie women from the east slope. Pure loneliness," Slim said sadly. "You can just see it in their eyes, like their only friend is that damn infernal wind."

"Mom wrote that Jep died last fall," Buddy said. Slim nodded. "What happened?"

"Just ran out of fuel, I suppose. After all, he was ninety something. One morning he just didn't come down to the lodge for breakfast, and when I went up to his cabin I found him dead in bed."

"Where did you bury him?"

"Didn't!" Slim said without inflection.

"What?!" Buddy was astonished.

"Nope, your daddy and me packed him back to that ridge above Cloud Lake and built him a Sioux burial platform. That was the way he wanted it."

"Poor old guy. Did he have any family?"

"Well, you, for one! You and your Daddy, and me and Ethel. There ain't one of us that ain't in Jep's debt. Hell, when I caught him poaching that spring, he could have left me and my gimped-up leg right there in that avalanche field to freeze to death, and nobody would have been the wiser. But not Jep. Nope, he helped me all the way back to Skyline, even though it meant he was headed straight into trouble with the law. *We* was his family, and he's just as much a part of your ancestry as if he were blood to you."

Buddy thought about Casey and Slim circumventing the process of death certificates and coroner's reports by simply taking Jep up to Cloud Lake. Somehow it was fitting. Not just because it was the Sioux custom, but because it was in keeping with his family ways.

"Buddy, stop!" the old man suddenly yelled. Buddy's foot leapt from the gas peddle onto the brake with such force that the Bronco skidded in the soft sand and rocked heavily onto two tires, threatening to roll over. The pursuant dust boiled around them. Without explanation, Slim swung open the door and lowered his brittle legs to the ground. Holding onto the fender for balance, he hobbled around the front of the Bronco. Buddy jumped out, not bothering to close the door, and ran around to catch Slim, thinking the old man was in pain. But Slim pushed him away.

"Don't you see it?" he exclaimed.

Buddy looked hard into the northern haze.

"No, it ain't out there." Slim stamped his foot on the ground, and little clouds of dust puffed up around his boots. "It's right here! We're standing on it." He turned to Buddy. "See how the land slopes away in every direction? I figure this must be the summit of the grade that train was pulling up when I hitched her. And judging by the lay of that mesa, I'll bet you a dollar to a doughnut that somewhere over yonder we'll find the railbed running like so." He swung his arm in a north-to-south arc. "Damn that infernal smoke. Without it, I could get a bead off the other mountain and in no time take us right to the spot where I cached that saddle."

Buddy took his binoculars from their case and began studying the desert. The late afternoon sun cast long shadows off legions of organ pipe and barrel cacti. The shadows cobwebbed across each other, forming an indigo netting that moulded to the contours of the desert floor. Then Buddy saw it—like water over a fall, the shadows pitched into a long, snake-back ravine.

"There's your arroyo, Grandpa." He pointed to the east.

Slim steadied himself against the Bronco door and trained the glasses where Buddy pointed. He looked for a long time, then he straightened and turned towards the mesa.

"Supposing that second mountain is back this way, and the railbed runs like so." He turned to the northwest. "Then the cache's got to be somewhere along that stretch yonder." He pointed to a particularly serpentine section of the ravine.

Buddy eased the Bronco off the dirt road and started cautiously across the desert floor, conscious that bouncing across the rough terrain would be painful for Slim. But the old man was too excited to consider turning back or even stopping for a rest. After about twenty minutes, they intersected a line straight as an arrow shaft across the desert and conspicuously void of mature cactus and mesquite. Again they stopped and got out.

"If my recollection serves me"—Slim looked up and down the railbed—"we got to go farther up that way to where the arroyo swings close to the railroad."

Buddy turned and looked the way they'd come, back towards the visible mesa. Suddenly he had an idea. Retrieving his polarized sunglasses from their case on the visor, he put them on and again studied the northern horizon. It worked. Backlit by the waning sun, the ghostly form of the second mesa appeared off the left shoulder of the first one. Now it was Buddy who was excited. He'd been afraid, even before he left Canada, that the old man's recall might be waning in its own sunset. But obviously, Slim's memory was doing just fine.

The iron rails had been pulled up long ago, and the road ties had rotted away, leaving a corrugated surface that heaved and pitched the Bronco far worse than the desert floor. But Slim, wearing the polarized glasses, focussed only on the position of the two mesas until finally the western cliff face on each peak came into line. And, just as Slim had predicted, the arroyo swung close to the railbed. They parked and walked to the ravine. Slim moved upstream twenty feet until the line of the mountains was exact with the picture in his memory.

"This is it!" Slim exclaimed. "This is the spot." He leaned over the edge of the bank, trying to see below the rim, but it was too undercut. "Buddy, take a rope and climb down to see what you see."

Buddy pulled a saddle rope from the equipment stashed in the back of the Bronco and tied one end to the Ford's bumper. Casting the coils out over the arroyo, he backed over the bank and rappelled below the edge. The gully was thirty feet deep and twice that distance in width. And judging by the fresh tangle of desert debris deposited high along the side walls, a flash flood had recently come through. There was a shelf a couple of feet wide, ten feet below the rim, on which Buddy could stand. He looked around, but he didn't see any evidence of caves. "How far below the rim was the cave?" he shouted.

"Ten, maybe fifteen feet," Slim yelled from above.

Buddy hiked on the shelf farther downstream, then upstream. Still there was nothing.

"I can't find it," Buddy called up to Slim. "It looks like maybe the bank has fallen in at some time. Maybe the cave's collapsed."

Slim stood and turned towards the two mesas, squinting through the dark glasses. He recalled the events of that day so long ago. "Nope," he said finally, "this is the place. You may have to do some digging, but I'm sure we're right on target."

"It's getting pretty late, Grandpa," Buddy said as he climbed out of the arroyo. "I think we should mark this spot and come back tomorrow." He brushed the dust from his Levi's. "We can drive back to Punto Lindo, get a motel room and come back early in the morning before the sun gets too hot."

"Sure, we *could* do that, but we could also camp right here. We got water and coffee and our bedrolls—I'd imagine we could get by without a couple of meals, don't you think?"

Buddy was against the idea. They'd have to sleep on the ground, and he knew that desert nights were bitter cold without ground vegetation to hold the warmth. It would be hard on the old man. Still, it was obviously what Slim wanted. So, taking a machete, Buddy lowered himself again into the ravine to collect firewood from the mesquite brush that grew along the wall—maybe the same clump Slim had hidden behind seventy years ago.

It was a symphony sunset. Shafts of crimson light trumpeted overhead, and kettledrum thunderheads boomed between the violin strains of night and the reed-thin flutes of wind sweeping across the desert. The pungent, oily smell of burning wood rose from the campfire, and its liquid light danced off the men's faces. While Buddy tended a blackened pot of boiling coffee grounds, Slim scrubbed a lariat with the back side of his hunting knife, causing the strands of jute to bristle like the spines on a hedgehog.

"We used to do this on the trail," Slim said, sitting on his bedroll with the rope coiled at his feet. "The old saddle tramps claimed snakes won't cross a burred rope cuz it scratches their bellies. Don't know if it's a fact, but I ain't yet shared my sleeping bag with a rattler."

Buddy poured the steaming brew into two tin cups and handed one to Slim, who moved nearer the fire and squatted on his haunches. Neither man spoke for some time. "How are things going for you in Canada, Buddy? Did you ever find your pilot friend?" Slim asked. "The guy who was working with you collaring those caribou?"

"Marc? No, not a trace of him or his plane. The north country's pretty unforgiving, and she hides her victims well."

Slim nodded. "Weren't so long ago that the whole West was unforgiving. Tested your mettle from the moment you got up to the time you laid out your bedroll. Now," Slim muttered, "a man would be hard-pressed to find a place to die alone."

Buddy winced, feeling uneasy with a distant memory of the spring Slim's saddle horse, Trudy, died trying to swim the river.

Slim blew the steam from his coffee cup. "You still tracking your caribou?" he asked.

"Well, the project's grown, Grandpa," Buddy said. "Now we've got radios on caribou, wolves, moose, mountain sheep. In fact, we just received a grant to collar a few grizzly."

"So what's your overall plan?"

"Well, our final goal is to use the radio collars to get an overview of what's happening to the whole system, how the animals are using the land and all. What we're after is baseline information about what's hanging out with what, and where, and at what time of year, that kind of stuff."

"You figure you're plowing virgin ground?" Slim smiled, looking into his coffee cup.

"What do you mean?"

"Just this. You ain't the first one to see these things, you know. The Indians knowed the ways of the animals thousands of years ago."

"True." Buddy laughed. "But they didn't write it down."

"What?" Slim looked up, amused. "You saying it ain't legal tender 'less it's written down? Anyway, the Indians had their reports, but they was legends and stories. That's the way they told the people about how things are with nature, how critters all depend upon each other and the likes." Slim paused. "Remember that Sioux story Jep used to tell? The one about the raven and the wolves?"

Buddy smiled. He'd just finished writing a wildlife article on wolf predation, and he had been reminded at the time about the raven story. As Jep told it, a raven who was jealous of the elks' beauty learned to imitate the bull elk's bugle, and one fall, he called the elk herds away to a distant land far from their traditional range. For the next two seasons, the raven danced across the sky, telling all who would listen of his unrivalled grandeur. But his friends the wolves, who before had shared so many meals with the raven, only became sadder and sadder, mourning the loss of the elk.

And with each passing year the size of the wolf pack dwindled as fewer and fewer pups were born. Moreover, to the raven's sorrow, he wasn't invited to eat with them, for the wolves didn't have enough for themselves. Finally the bird could bear it no longer, and he flew to the distant land and called the elk back to their home range. But the wolves didn't trust the raven at first, and only after a couple of seasons did the pack size begin to increase again.

Buddy's report wasn't nearly so rich and poetic. He'd concluded in his summation, "Wolf packs expand and decline in a direct, though delayed, correspondence to the abundance or absence of their prey."

"The problem is"—Slim shifted slightly on his haunches—"when it comes to studying nature, science tries to make things too exact when all along nature survives by chance and likelihood."

Again Buddy smiled at the old man's wisdom. "Biology, I must admit, tries to make exacting laws out of improbabilities. That grizzly grant we just got is a classic example. When we get through with our study, they'll expect us to come up with some definite conclusion, like grizzlies kill twenty per cent of all caribou calves. But you and I both know that, in fact, grizzlies kill one hundred per cent if they can and if the advantage is in their favour—and *none* when they can't."

Slim laughed. "I guess all I'm saying is that in some ways"—he looked across the fire at Buddy—"legends and stories are still good currency cuz they leave room for the unexpected."

The shrill spiked cry of an elf owl, perched on a nearby saguaro cactus, pierced the night. Suddenly Buddy sensed that the desert around them was alive and teeming with activity, even though he couldn't see it. For all of man's technological antennae, Buddy thought, they really saw so little, and understood far less. Maybe the Indians did know more.

"But let me ask you something straight, Buddy," Slim said, still studying his grandson's face across the fire. "Why does the government and these foundations pay so much money for your studies? Not that I'm saying they ain't worth it, but why all of a sudden are they so important?"

Buddy stared for a long time into the flames. "In a nutshell, Grandpa, we don't have time any more to learn in the way the Indians did. We've gotten too good at destroying our nest." He paused, carefully picking his words so the old man would understand.

"The hard truth is that every wildlife system in the world is on the edge of collapsing. In fact, a lot have already bit the biscuit because we've pulled their environment out from under them. What it boils down to is that man's changing the rules of nature even before we understand them. So, to answer your question, I guess that's the hurry, to discover nature's rules while they're still in operation."

"I guess I agree with what you're saying, son, but don't forget—we're all users." Slim rubbed his hands together and held them to the fire. "You come from a family that made its livelihood off wild animals. Your daddy and me was guides and hunters long before you was even born. Hell, you were raised on elk steaks and moose roasts."

"Grandpa, it's not the practice," Buddy interrupted, "it's the speed at which we're doing it. It's the rate of change. That's what's killing our nest. That's the problem—everything's happening so much faster nowadays!"

Both men watched the coals ebb and flare with the night breeze. "You know, Buddy, sitting here like this, around the fire and all"—Slim looked into the dark desert—"it don't seem like nothing's changed since I rode range here seventy years ago. Could be seventy years or even seven hundred years ago. But, son, I know maybe better than even you that there's a lot of truth in what you're saying." The old man drew a deep breath and released a sigh that would haunt Buddy for years. It was a sigh heavy and sad, and in it Buddy suddenly understood just how much change the old man had seen.

But Buddy also heard something else in Slim's sigh, something more fundamental. Something that cut deep into him. It was like an ancient wail, Buddy thought, the muted cry of a long lineage of Jep's ancestors, maybe even his own ancestors, their stories and legends reduced to mere whispers by the winds of change.

"It's getting late." The old man rose. "Let's turn in." Slim took the burred saddle rope and laid it in a circle around their bedrolls. "It'll be interesting to see if this works."

It will be interesting to see if this trip has just been a wild-goose chase, Buddy reflected as he lay looking up at the explosion of stars arching from horizon to horizon.

Buddy awoke just before dawn. He was delighted that no snakes had tried to share his bedroll. Already Slim was poking about in the fire pit, folding the coals around the coffeepot and fanning them with his hat. He seemed as impatient and anxious as a child on Christmas morning. Buddy suspected Slim hadn't slept all night. By the time they'd each had a cup of coffee, the sun caught the top of both mesas. When it was light enough to see, Buddy took a collapsible shovel and again rappelled over the bank, while Slim rocked impatiently on his heels on the rim.

Buddy wasn't sure where to start. But since the old man's directions had been pretty accurate so far, Buddy decided to begin digging right where Slim said. Two hours passed, then suddenly Buddy saw it fall from the shovel, a dull grey object about the size of a silver dollar. He let out a holler that rattled and echoed off the arroyo's walls. And soon he was up the rope with the object clenched in his right hand, waving it like he'd just discovered Spanish gold bullion.

"What you got, son?" Slim asked excitedly.

"It's a concho, off a saddle!"

Slim's grin spread across his face.

Buddy handed the silver disk to him and disappeared once

more over the bank. When he returned, he had three more conchos, a snaffle bit off a bridle, some cinch rings and the wooden tree of a saddle.

Looking at the treasures laid out on the desert floor, Buddy was filled with an overwhelming sense of destiny, of closing a circle seventy years in circumference.

"How could you be so sure after all those years?" he asked.

"By the story," Slim said. "The story was the map. Everything we needed to know was in there." Then he smiled, his ancient fingers touching each artifact delicately. "And now"—he rocked back and held Buddy in his eyes—"you can pack all of this up—and bury it right where you found it!"

Buddy's jaw dropped.

"That's right, put the conchos in a tobacco tin so they're easier to find the next time." Slim ignored Buddy's shocked expression.

Surely the old man was teasing him, Buddy thought, or maybe somehow testing him. But when he looked into Slim's eyes, Buddy saw that his grandfather meant every word. Buddy was confused. Still, he had too much respect for Slim's judgement to challenge it. Obediently, he rummaged around in the Bronco, finding only the Prince Albert can.

"What should I do with the dynamite caps?" he called.

"Leave 'em in the can with the conchos," Slim said, then laughed. "Who knows, someday somebody might need 'em to blow up that power station." He turned to the north and the brown haze that had again saturated the horizon. "No, wait, leave out a few and we'll shoot off that old dynamite before we cross back into Texas. No need risking a run-in with the law over a few old charges of gunpowder."

Buddy laid the conchos and bridle parts carefully in the tobacco can and snapped on the lid tightly. He wondered who might open it next. Collecting the rest of the saddle parts into a canvas bag, he descended once again into the arroyo.

When Buddy returned, Slim had walked a few hundred yards into the desert. He stood tall and straight, facing the sun. There was something commanding about the old man's silhouette. Like the dark outline of one of the mesas, immutable, interminable. The whole desert seemed to radiate away from the black form like a brilliant, blazing aura. As Buddy stood staring transfixed at Slim's outline seemingly on the cusp of becoming pure energy, he suddenly realized their journey had nothing to do with finding a lost saddle, never had.

"You know what doesn't change, Buddy?" The old man continued to face the sun as Buddy stepped up beside him. "The voice of our ancestors in the legends." He paused. "It's like Jep used to say: 'We carry our ancestors with us.' Their stories tell us not just who they were and where we come from, but in some measure, they tell us who we are. They show us our character, give us our confidence, our courage." Again Slim fell silent. Then he turned from the sun to his grandson.

"Bring your children here, and their children, in turn. Do like you and me done and show them how to take a bearing off those two mesas—show 'em how to find the arroyo and the saddle. But most of all, Buddy," he said, touching his grandson's hand, "tell them the stories."

On the way to the border, they stopped to detonate the dynamite that had been rolling around on the floor of the Bronco. Unfortunately, because the primer fuse linking the charges had been bent and kinked from years of abuse in the old Ford, the charges didn't go off sequentially, or for that matter simultaneously. And it wasn't until Slim and Buddy were well into Texas that the final charge shook the desert, and the blue and white sign toppled face first onto the rust-red sand.

PRINTED IN CANADA